Peter FitzSimons is a journalist with the *Sydney Morning Herald* and *Sun-Herald*, and a busy events and motivational speaker.

He is the author of more than thirty books, including *Tobruk, Kokoda, Batavia, Eureka, Ned Kelly, Gallipoli, Fromelles and Pozières, Victory at Villers-Bretonneux* and biographies of Douglas Mawson, Nancy Wake, Kim Beazley, Nick Farr-Jones, Les Darcy, Steve Waugh and John Eales, and is Australia's biggest selling narrative non-fiction author of the last twenty years.

Peter was named a Member of the Order of Australia for services to literature as a biographer, sports journalist and commentator, and to the community through contributions to conservation, disability care, social welfare and sporting organisations. He is also Chair of the Australian Republican Movement.

He lives with his wife, Lisa Wilkinson, and their three children in Sydney.

THE GREAT
AUSSIE BLOKE SLIM-DOWN

PETER FITZSIMONS

EBURY
PRESS

An Ebury Press book
Published by Penguin Random House Australia Pty Ltd
Level 3, 100 Pacific Highway, North Sydney NSW 2060
www.penguin.com.au

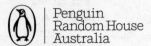

Penguin
Random House
Australia

First published by Ebury Press in 2016

Addresses for the Penguin Random House group of companies can be found at global.penguinrandomhouse.com/offices.

National Library of Australia
Cataloguing-in-Publication entry

FitzSimons, Peter, author
The great Aussie bloke slim-down: how an over-50 former footballer went from fat to fit . . . and lost 45 kilos/Peter FitzSimons

ISBN 978 0 14378 186 8 (paperback)

FitzSimons, Peter
Overweight men – Australia – Anecdotes
Ex-football players – Australia – Nutrition – Anecdotes
Weight loss – Australia – Biography – Anecdotes
Reducing diets – Anecdotes

305.31092

Cover photo by Peter Morris
Cover design by Christa Moffitt, Christabella Designs
Internal design and typesetting by Midland Typesetters, Australia
Printed in Australia by Griffin Press, an accredited ISO AS/NZS 14001:2004 Environmental Management System printer

Penguin Random House Australia uses papers that are natural, renewable and recyclable products and made from wood grown in sustainable forests. The logging and manufacturing processes are expected to conform to the environmental regulations of the country of origin.

To all the fat blokes out there who are jack of it –
had a gutful of having a gutful – and are finally intent
on getting on top of this. I seriously hope this book
helps. We can feel young and strong again!

Contents

Foreword

by Lisa Wilkinson

While I've always been proud of my husband and his writing, I am particularly proud of this book, and most especially the change in his life, and our marriage, that it documents.

For 25 years I have seen his weight go up and down, invariably, alas, with each *up* outdoing each *down* to the point that the 126 kilogram Wallaby second-rower I married in 1992, whose fighting weight had been 114 kilograms only two years earlier, had turned into 152 kilograms of a Whole-Lotta-Love by New Year's Day 2011.

And of course my broad experience has been matched by hundreds of thousands, let's say *millions*, of women across Australia, and it's been the case for decades. The problem is, what do you do in the face of it?

Nag? Encourage? Give him a gentle talking to, about how you want him to be around for another 50 years, not just another 20? I, frankly, tried all of those – and a couple of others besides – but with no luck. Being moderate in anything is just not in Pete's nature, which, when applied to most things like familial love, work ethic, sport, romance, fatherhood, the Australian republic and having fun, made me fall in love with him in the first place. But not in the eating.

And then there was the drinking.

To be fair, Pete was not a bad man with too much grog in him.

But he was *not* the man I married. When he drank too much, he became careless of those around him, careless in his judgement, careless in the way he spoke to me, his fuse was shorter, his parenting and partnering so much less energetic, and he was generally much less fun to be around.

Pete never drank at home for the first 15 years of our marriage, but the pressures of book deadlines, of daily journalism, of parenting and his professional speaking commitments, which could involve lunches and dinners as often as four times a week, conspired to mean that knocking back copious amounts of alcohol became part of his life, at home as well.

There were periods when he realised what he was doing, stopped – ceased both eating and drinking to excess, lost weight – and everything suddenly got better.

But the minute he got to his target weight and proved that he could do it, figured he had this whole weight loss, non-drinking thing tapped, he fell into the old trap of going back to living his old life – pass-the-pies and pull-the-cork-out-please – and the weight quickly piled back on.

Every time we talked about it, I'd end up getting precisely nowhere. He'd promise to pull back, and might for a short time, but soon he'd be back to his old over-indulgent lifestyle. Until, one day, it was like a light went on, like all the planets suddenly aligned and he worked it out. He worked out how to live the full life he does, always at a million miles an hour, and enjoy it every bit as much as he ever did and more, *without* over-indulging, without the stress on our relationship, his heart, or even his belt buckle. And it wasn't me, it was a simple conversation with a mate that did it. (Thanks, Jordan.)

Ultimately I hope *The Great Aussie Bloke Slim-Down* will be that for the men who read this book – a chat with a mate they can trust, a catalyst for positive change.

It has taken me a while, frankly, to believe that Pete's latest commitment to losing weight was not just one more passing phase, that he wasn't going to revert to the old ways, but, two years in, I am now convinced.

I have a new man on my hands, and in my arms . . .

He is just like the old man, but lighter, younger, faster, more patient, more fun. And an even better father than he was.

I do hope this book might have a similarly beneficial effect on your partner.

Warmest regards,
Lisa Wilkinson,
Sydney, September 2016

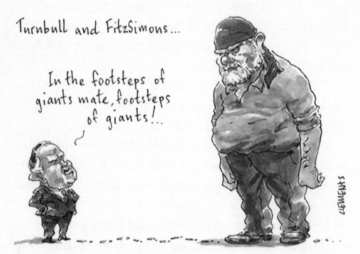

The cartoonists were *most* unkind when I took over as Chair of the Australian Republican Movement. (Rod Clement)

Introduction

Oi! You. Fatty Boomka. Yes, you.

Don't look around at others. I am talking to you, bloke. And don't be offended at being called Fatty Boomka either, precious, because I used to *be* you. You and I were the Boomka twins, and I could more than hold my own against you on the other end of the seesaw. And, just like you, my weight yo-yoed up and down for 30 odd years, with the problem being that the low point of every downward yo kept trending upwards, as did the high yo.

Oh, come on. You have been on exactly the same yo-yo weight plan – *very fat . . . pretty fat . . . not-so-fat-but-still-a-whole-lot-to-love . . . VERY bloody fat* – and we both know it.

Now, before you and I continue, I need to make a couple of things clear:

I am in no way a nutritional expert, but I respect those who are.

I am not an expert on human movement.

I am as far from an academic as it gets.

I really am *you*, Boomka.

I have faced exactly the same expanding waistline challenges as you, elbowed you out of the way at the buffet table, staggered past you at the bar, disgraced myself at Aunty Mary's with a notorious display of how many extra helpings of dessert just one man could have, eaten more sneaky Kit Kats than you when our wives weren't looking and, most significantly, suffered alongside you every New Year's Day when we both stepped on our bathroom scales to work out just how bad the damage had been over the last 12 months.

For yonks, mate, while standing on those scales, just like you, I'd breathe out heavily to get rid of all that weighty oxygen, then tucked my tummy in 'cos that just might help, then I'd lean out to the right, just like you did, and manage to make them read about two kilos lighter, just like you did . . .

How am I going? Do you accept now, that I *am* you?

And then, of course, digital scales came along and *ruined everything* for us, didn't they? (Well, nearly. I still fancy myself as something of a 'scales whisperer', lowering myself gently while holding on to the shower stall so as not to frighten it high, before removing my hand. By talking to the scales gently, rocking back a little and lifting my left and right toe at the same time, I can STILL lop about .3 of a kilo off.)

Still, back then, we didn't truly care, did we, mate? 'Cos despite making fabulous New Year's resolutions on

1 January with you, about how this year we were *really* going to get back into shape, we both know what happened. For I was with you on 3 January, too, when we both decided to break all those resolutions anyway, and get back to our regular eating and drinking patterns.

Pass the pies, son! And the wine! And the beer! Double portions, fer Chrissakes. We have *three* days of health-nut dieting madness to make up for! New Year's resolutions are for wusses, anyway.

And so, as the days grew cold, and we grew old, we just kept getting bigger and bigger, am I right? They say that inside every fat man there is a thin man trying to get out, but more to the point, there is also a somewhat confused older man, wondering on a wan night as the owls hoot in the distance and the lost and lonely freight train struggles slowly and painfully up yonder hill, just where the younger, fitter, stronger man he used to be . . . bloody well *went*, and how did it get to this?

Depressing, sometimes, wasn't it? Christ. Pass some more pies, son, and let's get pissed again. *That*'ll make us feel better.

And it always did.

Until the next morning, when the original problem was inevitably worse.

But, seriously, mate, this time, take pause. Put down the party pie. I repeat. Put *down* the party pie. Now, put your hands over your head, and move away from the plate. I've got you covered.

Focus!

3

Now, though I have been with you every step of the way on this journey, if this intro tells you anything, it is to let you know, Boomka, that I have turned back. I am sick of this tedious trudging up the mountain of our own weight, getting slower and slower, ever more exhausted, and feeling older than our years, haunted by the vision of fat mates falling into the abyss, never to return . . .

I've gone back the other way. And I want you to follow in my sylph-like footsteps!

For you see, I reckon I have cracked the code. I have worked this bastard out, so it won't bother us anymore.

To repeat, I don't claim, remotely, to be an expert on weight-loss programs. But I know you and the way you think.

(You are still thinking about the party pies, aren't you? See? When it comes to Boomka brainwaves, I am so tuned in to your station it's *not true*!)

And so from now, I'm establishing the 'yo diet', which is totally different to all the rest we've tried, and failed at.

See, the problem with all those diets was that we were just following them, and yes, seeing some results, but not actually learning anything. We didn't know more at the end of the diet than we did at the beginning, and so quickly went back to our old ways.

With the help of experts – some of whom speak complicated gibberish, but which I've translated into the fluent 'Aussie bloke' I've been mastering for donkey's years – I've worked out how to get my weight down so it bloody well stays down, and live a whole lot healthier life to boot.

The best thing is, it works for others, too.

When I wrote an article for the *Sydney Morning Herald* for New Year's Day 2016 about my experience of dropping 30 kilos – which is now 42 kilos, as of mid-September – it not only went viral, but ever since I have been accosted, I kid you not, by blokes in airports, restaurants and on the street, at the footy, often with beaming wives, telling me and often my wife too how that article changed their lives and that they've finally dropped an untold number of kilos, with more ease than they ever thought possible. The emails have also flooded in, all saying that for the first time in their lives they had dropped heaps of kilos *without going hungry*. With that sort of reaction from just one article, my publishers were quick to agree there was a book in it. And here it is!

So do you want to hear the answer, or not? Bloke to bloke, no bullshit? This is not about 'fat-shaming', a phrase in vogue right now. Lots of blokes are overweight, and quite happy to be so. Good luck to them. But heaps more are jack of carrying way too much pud, and they want the form and energy of their youth back. They're looking for a solution, without the crap. Does that sound like you?

Read on, you champion.

To begin, let's review the journey you and I have been on so far.

ONE

Gawd almighty, how did we get this fat in the first place?

'I'm on the sea-food diet. I sees food, I eats it.'
George Foreman, in an interview with me, in Sydney, 2003

'Ask not what you can do for your country. Ask what's for lunch.'
Orson Welles, actor, writer, director and famous fat man

'Most of what we're consuming today is no longer, strictly speaking, food at all, and how we're consuming it – in the car, in front of the TV, and increasingly alone – is not really eating.'
Michael Pollan, American health guru

There's a scene I love in *M*A*S*H*, where Hawkeye is trying to lift the spirits of a soldier who has just lost his leg in a battle. The soldier's lying in bed, trying to gather himself to face life again.

Very roughly, and from memory only – oh, do get nicked, you pedantic *M*A*S*H* nutters – it goes something like this . . .

'Say, where you from, soldier?' Hawkeye asks brightly.

'Bettsville, Ohio,' the soldier replies.

'*Bettsville*, Ohio?' Hawkeye says. 'Isn't that where the kids drag Main every day before and after school? Where the local baseball team just about made the finals a few years back, only to miss out because of some crazy umpiring decisions at the last hurdle. Bettsville, Ohio . . . doesn't that have, right on the edge of town, a hamburger joint that makes the best hamburgers and greasiest, most delicious French fries in the whole state?'

'That's Bettsville!' the soldier cries excitedly. 'You've been there!'

'No,' Hawkeye replies. 'But I grew up in the same small town in Maine.'

Boom boom, Boomka!

Which brings me to our own more-or-less common experience.

In my case, I was so big as a newborn baby that I set a record with my 25½ inch length – Mum always said, 'Petey-boy, you were so long, you were born on the 27th, the 28th and the 29th June 1961.'

In your case, I'm guessing you were not that long, but still good on the tooth, right?

We just kept eating like ravenous dingo cubs from the first, *and* kept growing. In my case, at the age of 14, I had grown so much that the river of hand-me-downs that had been flowing from my bevy of older, bigger brothers, suddenly turned. For the first time, they began to wear clothes that I was growing out of.

Sometimes we had to change clothes straight after breakfast, as the buttons started to pop. And *then* I hit puberty!

Of course my weight kept soaring, but so did my height. And weren't we all much the same?

You and I were blessed to be raised in a country where, generally, there was never an issue with not having enough food on the table. Growing up, up, up, there was never any problem with getting fat because though we were eating like horses, and putting on *heaps* of weight, it didn't matter because we were also getting taller. And we were actually moving. Being born in the pre-Internet age, we didn't 'virtually' live, we *lived*, and walked and ran and jumped and climbed and played games that required our limbs to move.

For those like me, getting particularly tall, we could eat for Australia and still there was no problem in early adulthood. Because in our 20s, we were still fit and active, so it didn't matter so much if we were big.

For me, it was a tad embarrassing at Wallaby fitness tests; all the other guys would climb onto the ordinary scales while Alan Jones and then Bob Dwyer would send Tommy Lawton and me – still breathing in and leaning waaaay out to the right, hoping against hope – down to the scales they used for the cows at the abattoirs.

But, what the hell?

We were still running around, so it didn't matter. I was, in fact, running around well enough and fast enough that in 1990 when *60 Minutes* did a story on 'Who Is Austra-lia's Fittest Athlete?' I was even winning after five of the eight events, finally coming in fourth behind the likes of Ironmen Guy Leech and Grant Kenny. I even managed to beat Olympic gold medal swimmer Duncan Armstrong and famed runner Andrew Lloyd. (If you care, then google: *60 Minutes,* Australia's Fittest Athlete.)

The true problem for most of us started in our early 30s and went on from there as we became so much less physic-ally active, and much more focused on careers, kids of our own, working for the man and paying the rent. But that was happening to so many blokes around us at the same time that it became *normal* to be thickset, just like everyone else.

Hence, the problem. Our lives had changed, but our eating habits had not.

And there were so many of us in the same boat sinking below the Plimsoll line that being fat became, if not the new black, at least the new normal.

So, early on, being on the cuddly side of things didn't particularly bother us.

Because, just like everyone else, though less physically active, we still kept reaching for the extra party pies with sauce, the extra beer, the second helpings of apple pie. Just as we always had.

Because that's the sort of Aussie bloke we are, am I right?

Diets? We'd heard of them, but really didn't like the sound of them. There was something so very . . . unmanly about them. The only diet tip we ever followed was the one provided by Miss Piggy: 'Never eat anything you can't lift.'

Again, true, a few mates of ours didn't get big like us. And other mates of theirs were out and out – what's that word again? – *wankers.*

They were health nuts, who did things like:

- Went to the gym. (They actually paid money for this! Handed over the readies, just to do P.E. when no-one was forcing them to, like in school! Weirdos. DANGEROUS weirdos!)
- Didn't eat the fat and rind on their five slices of bacon at breakfast. (Seriously, who DOES that? It was my firm view that even cutting off the rind was the surest tell-tale sign of the lot that you were that most unspeakable of all things, a 'health nut'.)
- Pushed the dessert plate away and said, 'Oh, no, I couldn't possibly have another slice . . .' (ACTUAL men with testosterone in them said this! We know pretending to be full is compulsory female behaviour, but these were people who, technically, were presumed to stand up as they pissed!)
- Exercised regularly – not to bash some bastard coming the other way, like we did in football, like normal blokes did, but – just for the SAKE of exercise!
- Used new-fangled and incomprehensible terms like 'protein', 'cardiovascular exercise' and 'I'll do the washing up'.
- Proudly still fitted into their wedding suit, as long as five years after the big day. (Yes, they were married

and still fit! Did they miss the point of the ceremony? Love, honour and let yourself go, it's the Australian way. #STRAYA!)

- Had two beers and *only* two. Sometimes even none!
- Ate green leaves with lunch or dinner by CHOICE – not by accident while trying to shovel steak and chips into their gobs.
- Declared themselves to be *vegetarians*. Bloody hell. Look, we didn't mind vegetarians per se, but just weren't convinced we could eat a whole one.
- Went to the 'fresh produce' (Editor, am I spelling that correctly?) section of the supermarket before the potato chip section. (Let's face it. Weren't you and I only ever in the fresh produce section because we got to see potatoes in their repulsive natural state before they got cut up and thrown in a deep fryer, to either come to us as hot chippies, or the haute cuisine of . . . salt and vinegar chips?)

Listen, they also tended to be blokes who were '*in touch with their feelings*' – say no more. All of that was not for us. Blokes like that were dead-set weird, and simply not P.L.U. (People Like Us).

And, yes, our gut looked big in that, but so what? Every other bastard we knew our age, or at least most blokes we hung around with, had a big gut, too, and besides which, it didn't look *that* big!

And herein lies the historical essence of our problem. You and me, mate . . .

All our lives, we have suffered from *high* self-esteem. You will recall that book, *Men are from Mars, Women are from Venus*, the central premise being that men and women are just wired differently and look at everything in different ways.

When it comes to our weights, there is an obvious truth to that.

Even when our darlings have been at their most svelte, they have never emerged from the shower to look at themselves naked in the mirror with anything less than one eyebrow raised, as they see too much weight on their thighs, their hips, their tummies.

Well, not us, and certainly not me.

Without a word of a lie, even when I reached 152 kilograms – and the only difference between me and a whale was a pair of underpants and a beard – I would emerge from the shower, look at myself in the mirror, and see nothing less than . . . a FINE FIGURE OF A MAN!

You, too?

Robust, yes, but in a *good* way. (And if I flexed and the steam level was right, I looked almost dangerously good. Particularly the upper torso. *Is it too late to be a professional body builder?* I would idly wonder. Never, if I added more steam. And if I held my breath and tucked my tummy in, I could even get away without too much steam.)

Look, I guess by one reckoning, the front of my torso actually looked like a hairy mudslide, with waves of billowing fat cascading down to where I guess my groin must have been, but . . .

But, I reckon I had a nice personality, and that was the main thing. And I really didn't *see* the hairy mudslide, anyway.

I innately knew that Lisa was lucky to have me.

And so we just kept getting bigger as the years went by. Sure we'd get serious for a bit, and the weight would go down, but then we'd get to Christmas and what kind of *dickhead* doesn't have extra helpings of turkey and pudding on Christmas Day, not to mention getting pissed as a newt on New Year's Eve? And then there was your mate's birthday drinks a week later, not to forget the Australia Day holidays and . . .

And before we knew it, we were back to living just the way we always did, only a little heavier, which reminds me, love, is there something wrong with that washing powder we are using because I swear all my clothes have been getting tighter and smaller lately, you know?

And, of course, it really wasn't just you and me and our mates.

Over the last quarter of a century, the average weight of Australian men has increased by 6.5 kilograms – about a stone in the old money – and we now tip the scales at an average of 85.9 kilograms. (I know. That still sounds downright *emaciated* to me, too, but that is just how far you and I have come on our journey up fat mountain.) And women are running us close, with an increase of 5.7 kilograms in that time, to now weigh an average of 71 kilograms.[1]

But here's the thing.

It is actually no laughing matter.

It's *killing* us.

The Australian Institute of Health and Welfare reported in 2014 that nine out of ten people currently on their death beds are there because of chronic illnesses, ranging from heart disease to cancer to Type 2 diabetes.[2]

And here's the thing. ALL OF THOSE can be directly linked to obesity and dangerous eating habits.

And while you really do see heaps of badly overweight men in their 40s, 50s and 60s, you don't see nearly as many in their late 70s and 80s, because the bitter truth is if they haven't got their weight under control by that time, they mostly . . . *die.*

I know that's a bit brutal, just saying it like that. But if nothing else makes you understand that this is serious, that we all have to concentrate, surely that alone is worth thinking about?

Most tragic, of course, is the reality that the obesity epidemic is not even restricted to men and women in our age group. As they watch us eat and follow our lead, a quarter of our kids are overweight or obese, while just nudging towards two-thirds of the whole adult population is overweight.

What the hell happened to us, Australia?

We all know the image of the Man from Snowy River, '*racing down the mountain like a torrent down its bed*', of the Australian soldiers storming ashore and up to the heights of Gallipoli, of *Ashes to Ashes, dust to dust, if Lillee don't get 'em, Thommo must,* of being a race of bronzed Aussie lifesavers, with rippling muscles and granite jaws.

Today, the horse would probably buckle under the weight of the Man from Snowy River. And we'd be buggered if someone told us to try and climb *those* cliffs!

Ashes to Ashes, dust to dust, we can fit into our trousers, but only just.

We were a hardy, lean, athletic people.

These days we make the list of the Top Five Fattest Nations – at least in the front-line of the developed world – on Earth! We're not in control of the calories that come to our beer guts or the manner in which they come. We drive our kids to school, even when it's less than a kilometre away. And while *it's a long way to the shop if you want a sausage roll*, it ain't so far if you take two tonnes of machinery out on the road to go and get it – as most of us do.

Sure, when it comes to both slothfulness and obesity, we are not yet quite as fat as the Yanks, but that's just like saying Clive Palmer is probably not as annoying as Donald Trump.

Mate, you, me, all of us, as individuals and as a people, have got to get on top of this. Otherwise we will be under the dirt, in the extra-wide comfy coffin, much faster than we think.

TWO

Your 'Come to Jesus' moment (because you look like Buddha)

'Seize the moment. Remember all those women on the
Titanic who waved off the dessert cart.'
Erma Bombeck, humorist

'Everything you see I owe to spaghetti.'
Sophia Loren, actress
(Fair enough, but I suspect we could say the same of
Luciano Pavarotti?)

There are two major possibilities as to why you now have
this book in your hands.

Either you've dinkum had a 'Come to Jesus' moment
and realised that all the bullshit has to stop and you need
to nail this problem to the wall, or someone who loves you
wants you to have that moment, and hopes this book will

16

kickstart it. ('Bloody hell, if that stupid bastard in the red bandana can do it, clearly anyone can!')

One way or another, it has to be *you* who drives the whole thing or we are all wasting our time having you read on.

For many of us, the 'Come to Jesus' moment was a long time coming, and there were a few crucial steps along the way . . .

For me, the first step came when I was walking the Kokoda Track in 2002.

It was the hardest thing, physically, I've ever done, and that includes having eight All Blacks tap dance on my back when I was lying over the ball – and too often when I wasn't. Seriously, those bastards used to line up to carve their initials or their whole names on the back of my thighs. I can still see the one from Richard Loe which, not surprisingly, is misspelt. And I am tragically proud – *proud* do you hear me? – of being the only Wallaby in history, ever, sent from the field in a match against the All Blacks for violence! But I digress . . .

At least those Test matches only lasted for 80 minutes at a time.

Kokoda went on for damn nigh a week of agony! To this day, I am told, I am the second heaviest man to get across it in under six days. I started at 131 kilograms, and finished it at 126 kilograms.

The heaviest man across on record was the famed Wallaby prop, Chris 'Buddha' Handy, at 140 kilograms. Before starting out, the native porters eyed him warily, and then handed him a shovel. When he asked what it was for, they said, 'U E DI MIPELA NOR KALIM U.' Translated, it means, 'Because if you drop dead, big boy, *we* ain't carrying you out.'

At least the agony of walking Kokoda was enough to make me get healthier on one count. Prior to that, I had laboured under the idea that I could enjoy smoking moderately. But the way it turned out, I would smoke heavily on a Saturday night . . . sometimes stretching to Tuesday . . . and more often than not stretching into October.

Of course I gave up dozens of times, and equally took it up again dozens of times, plus one. It was always in a moment of weakness when I would just have a quick drag of someone's ciggie, cadge one, carry one, dot three, subtract two, buy a packet, and then be back on it again!

But it was while I was hauling my weary arse up to one of the highest summits of all on the Track, Brigade Hill, with my lungs burning, my legs feeling like lead weights, my spirit sinking fast, that the realisation struck me: I am no more bullet-proof as a bloke than were the brave Diggers who first trekked these parts to take on the Japanese heading to Port Moresby. Many of them died, as Eric Bogle sang of other Diggers, *quick and clean*. But if I didn't stop smoking that would not be my fate, I realised, it would be *slow and obscene*.

Somehow or other, the agony of that experience made me get it:

First, I was going to die a miserable death earlier than I otherwise would, if I didn't stop.

Second, the key realisation came – moderation was just not in me. If, once back in Australia, I had even one puff, I'd inevitably have two puffs, and it would be piss-weak not to finish the whole ciggie. And if you can have one ciggie, why not two and indeed why not the whole packet? And the whole wretched process would go on, as before.

Third, I had to stop, *cold*. And I did. Not only have I never smoked again, I've never been remotely tempted to.

Come to Jesus!

Two years later, I went through a remarkably similar experience with coffee. I was drinking so much of it, it was actually making me ill. Fifteen cups on a bad day! So I stopped. Cold. And have never been tempted to have it again.

Somehow or other, though, when it came to eating everything within cooee and drinking grog, the same solution never occurred to me, and I just kept going, getting ever bigger, until about five years ago, Lisa said to me outright, 'Pete, you're too heavy.'

At least I *think* it was her and I *think* that's what she said. At the very least, there was a certain muffled voice just like hers, coming from somewhere way beneath me, and it said something a lot like that.

I checked, and by gawd, she was right!

From my weight of 114 kilograms playing Test rugby – I know, I know, I'll have to tell you about it sometime – I had gone up to 152 kilograms, and was now living the miserable cliché of the formerly-fit-footballer-turned-to-fat. Sure, I had gone up and down many times as I got serious about my weight and then serious about chocolate cake and then serious about my weight again, but this was a post-war high. Lisa had a point.

Which is more than I had, as I was almost entirely curved. My belt was the sole reminder of where my waist used to be. I was big. Not Marlon Brando big, but I could definitely have auditioned to play him during the post-*Apocalypse Now* era.

No, I didn't act immediately, but it was the moment I truly realised that this was out of hand, and I had to get it in hand, before my hands got too big and my wedding ring cut off blood circulation to at least one finger. I loved my life and wanted more of it. But at that weight, at the age of 50, it was obvious I was a heart attack on legs on a countdown to let-down. (Perhaps just like my dad died, with his boots on, but dead before he hit the ground, on the family farm.)

Most other blokes who've got serious about their weight have had such moments. One I know of was with his mates on a drunken holiday in Bali when he emerged from a bar late at night, caught sight of himself in a shop window and stopped stock-still as they rampaged off down the street. *Is that me? That fat bloke staring back at me? How did I get to be this huuuge? What happened to me?* The bloke got serious, didn't drink a drop from that moment, came home, went to the gym, and has now become a qualified fitness instructor. One of his virtues is that he understands the headspace of the overweight clients he helps. For another bloke it was seeing a photo of himself on the dance floor at a wedding. It was not a photo of the pleasantly cuddly fellow he had imagined himself to be at the time. It was of a huge drunk man cavorting dangerously while other guests scattered wildly, the way farmyard chickens do before a crazy pig with a thorn between its toes. He, too, has now shed 30 per cent of his body weight.

Again, on the reckoning you've had your own moment, and are interested in the solutions, there are still a few things you need to know to properly understand them – even if I do take something of a Dennis Lillee run-up to get to the gravy.

For there is a story I have long cherished, about the time a famous European conductor visited Sydney just after the Second World War, to put our best and brightest orchestra through its paces. After just two minutes of the first practice, however, stricken by what he had heard, he called for silence. Holding up an instrument he took from the nearest musician, he said in his thickest Continental accent, 'Let us start from the beginning. This . . . well, this is called a violin.'

Which brings us, Boomka, to this thing called a 'balanced diet'.

For who the hell knows what that is, am I right? Every week brings new reports of what you should and shouldn't be eating, what the must-have-foods are and the must-not-have-foods, and they frequently contradict each other.

And I know I have not been alone in feeling confused.

So, you'll excuse me if, in this book, I pursue the same principle as I do in all my other books – and use my own ignorance as a tool. That is, when starting out to write military books like *Kokoda*, *Tobruk* and *Gallipoli*, it occurred to me that if I wasn't quite sure how many soldiers there were in a Platoon/Company/Battalion/Division, and whether a Sergeant-Major or a Lieutenant had more clout, it was a fair bet that a lot of my readers would be equally foggy . . . and so I have always built such basic information into my accounts.

So maybe *you* understand the difference between carbohydrate, protein and fats – and how much you need of them all in a balanced diet – but, trust me, a lot of blokes don't. And just as you have a working knowledge of how your car works – and the kind of fuel and oil it takes – for the guts of this book to work on *your* guts, you equally need to have a working knowledge of how your whole body works and the fuel it is designed to burn for maximum efficiency.

Very broadly, a food with a lot of **carbohydrate** in it is one that the body can easily break down into lots of sugars to give your body the energy it needs to function smoothly. Our body breaks the carbs down, or metabolises them if you will, into **glucose**, which, flowing through our blood, is our primary fuel, our main source of energy.

Examples where carbohydrates are found naturally are apples, broccoli, pears, bananas and potatoes. Equally broadly, the more fibre in them, the slower the body is to break it down, and the more evenly and naturally the glucose is released into the bloodstream.

Most processed foods, however, tend to be ones where the sugar has been added in bulk, while fibre has been decreased. And that sugar – which is just like the common table sugar known as sucrose that you and I used to add on top of our Weet-Bix – is composed of two basic parts. One half is pure glucose – meaning that part of sugar hits your bloodstream all but immediately, with no need of being gradually processed into glucose like natural food – and the other half is fructose or 'fruit sugar', an addictive substance twice as sweet as the glucose. (Cue, comedian: *'And that's when the trouble started . . .'*) But, we'll get to that!

Proteins, on the other hand, are what builds our muscles, our ligaments, our tendons, our hair and skin, etc. (It's actually a lot more complicated than that, and you also need proteins to move oxygen, minerals and vitamins around, not to mention produce hormones, but it's too dull and complicated to go into too deeply. I care no more about that ultra-refined part of it than I care how the fuel injection system of my car works. So long as it *does* work, I have no further questions. And I'll bet you feel the same. You and I need the *basics*, son, and the rest can sort itself.)

And then there are the **fats** of course, which you and I know only too well. Physiologically, we need good fats as opposed to bad fats, as a secondary, slower-to-burn source of energy – a reserve tank when no carbs are available – and they also have a role in helping vitamins become absorbed by the human body, including vitamins A, D, E and K . . . which, trust me, we all need.

The point is that one of the greatest problems in dealing with proper nutritional info is that 'fat', a normal part of many foods and one that we actually need, is exactly the same word which we use as an adjective to describe people like my mate Merv Hughes on a bad day – as in, 'He's *very* fat.'

(Gawd I miss the days when great cricketers were fat. Mark 'Tubby' Taylor, Beefy Botham, Shane Warne – but more on him, later. All gone with the wind and the rowing machine. Sigh. Now only the occasional golfer can be fat and it makes the average bloke's sports fantasy life much more restricting. At least we still have the odd Wallaby front-rower. Anyway, back to the fat.)

It means people make the mistake of automatically thinking fat = bad.

But fat is a lot more complicated than just that beautiful stuff that falls off your chops and bacon. There are animal fats and plant fats. Traditionally, it has been thought the animal fats are the baddies, and plant fats the goodies – hence why margarine became popular, as it was made from plant fats. Again, it gets complicated enough to kill a brown dog from this point and you'll be pleased to hear we don't need to go into it that deeply.

The main thing you need to know is that fat in food is not automatically bad – but ingesting huge quantities of it is. (And the same applies to carbs and protein, of course. It is that whole thing about balance.)

For now, understand that when you eat a meal or take a drink, your body works to break it all down, so as to take from it what it needs to have energy, stay healthy and simply function. Most interesting is what happens to the carbs, which go through a whole series of metabolic processes to finish as **glucose**, which is a form of sugar, and they then enter the bloodstream. To get those glucose molecules to where they are needed, the **pancreas** produces the hormone **insulin**, which sends the signals to the cells in muscles and organs where they are needed, to absorb the glucose so it can be used immediately for energy, thus helping remove it from the bloodstream. What happens to the excess glucose that is not needed on the spot?

Well, herein is the nub of the whole thing. First, excess glucose is converted into a substance called **glycogen**, of which 150 grams all up can be stored in the liver – providing us with about 24 hours of carbs energy – but after that, the excess is stored as fat.

So what happened to you and me, my fat friend, that made us get so damn BIG?

Clearly our diet – at least what we whacked in our gob, and poured down our throat – was waaaay out of kilter in this department.

I can't speak for you, but I can say that in my experience – and that of many Australian men – what blew me out beyond too much fat and too much alcohol, is too much sugar. Again, we'll get into that subject heavily a bit further down the track winding back, but before we do . . .

Let me put that another way: WE CONSUME TOO MUCH SUGAR.

And once again, Hercule Poirot style, 'The guilty party is . . . *dramatic pause* . . . Sugar!'

Bill Clinton, 1992 campaign style, 'It's the sugar, stupid!'

Mick Jagger, 'Brown Sugar!'

This is the key thing you need to understand:

When our body is looking for fuel, it first burns up the carbs, next it burns up the fat, and finally it burns the protein. The whole thing is organised by our **liver** following, among other things, the signals sent out by the aforementioned hormones. The more of the appetite-suppressing hormone **insulin** we have, which is released by ingested carbs, the less inclined we are to go on eating.

Our fat cells meanwhile, sensing the elevated level of glucose, release another hormone known as **leptin**. The fatter we are, the more fat cells we have, and so the more leptin is released, and our overall appetite is suppressed accordingly as our brain gets the message: 'Oi. We've got too much fat already. Stop eating so much.'

Is that neat, or is that *neat*?

It is NEAT!

It is almost enough to make me believe the religious nutters have been right about Intelligent Design all along, and everything is so intricately perfect that the only explanation is it *must* have come from God! It is *almost* enough to make me want to stand on an upturned fruit box on the corner of Pitt and Park streets myself, with a Bible in my hand, and shout to the passers-by that we *must* have been put here by a Supreme Being and all the ills of the world really are here, as they say, because 'a woman made out of one rib bone and a mound of dirt was tricked into eating fruit from a magical tree by a talking snake'!

Either that, or Charles Darwin spoke the truth. Either way, it really is fabulously balanced, and engineered to a 't'.

Anyway, very broadly, insulin sorts out our immediate hunger issues according to the glucose in our blood. It gives us the signals as to how much to put on our plate, and whether we want a second helping, while leptin is proportional to how much fat we are carrying and turns our overall appetite up or down accordingly.

Are you still with me, tree-people? God bless you, 'cos I'm singing for you, too.

So the last time you and I had a big night on the turps, complete with chippies, party pies and chocolate bars, all of it washed down by hot dogs at Harry's Cafe de Wheels at 3 am, we have put more sugars, fats and alcohol into our system than we could possibly burn up. So, what happens to the sugars, fats and alcohol we don't burn? It turns into fat stores, mostly around our bellies. You get it?

You remember in geography, how Wally Walmuth would say *blah, blah, blah*, the highest mountain range in the world is the Himalayas *blah, blah, blah* and the only thing you could remember afterwards was that one salient fact between the endless blahs? Well, this is like that. Get ready to *concentrate* now.

Blah, blah, blah . . .

Our tummy is designed as the main fuel tank of fixed size, while the fat that goes around it, and elsewhere over our body, is the rubbery reserve tank. But when we put too much dud fuel in the main tank, it keeps spilling over into the reserve tank, and that rubbery reserve tank just keeps getting bigger and bigger. And unlike a cool 1980s action movie where the car would just explode as Bruce Willis

27

smiled smugly from a distance and that would be it, our fat reserves just keep growing, the more fuel we pour in that is not burned up.

Die Hard and die slow, for so many of us, because we're taking in too much sugar, for starters.

Blah, blah, blah . . .

The point is that with sugar in the fuel, it sets up this extraordinarily self-perpetuating *vicious cycle*, until . . . we're going to need a bigger boat. And bigger shirts. And bigger pants.

So how do we get rid of those fat stores?

We change the fuel, mate, and put less in the tank.

If we lower the sugar-laden carbs – both as a proportion and in net quantity – after the body burns up the carbs, it has to burn up our fat stores and we get thinner, or at least, less fat. There will be endless nit-picking around the scientific edges of all this – trust me, I know – but this is the broad thrust of it. And you don't need much more than the broad thrust, a model in our head to work from.

I do hope it is all coming clearer now.

That's how, at his height, Arnold Schwarzenegger turned into what Clive James felicitously described as a 'brown condom stuffed with walnuts'. Arnie's diet and exercise regimen was precisely balanced to feed his muscle growth, while burning up nearly all the fat covering that muscle.

Now, if you take it to extremes, like my erstwhile biographical subject Douglas Mawson, and go on a starvation diet – in his case, forced upon him because he set a new record in Antarctica for being 'fucked and far from home', when, 200 miles from base, he lost 80 per cent of his supplies – your body starts to eat its own muscle. Again, we don't need to go there. (Though I can't resist adding that the finest polar explorer of the lot, Sir Ernest Shackleton, deliberately fattened himself up before going on his massive treks – 'One thus acquires a layer of fat all over in much the same way [as] the indigenous fauna of these latitudes' – specifically so he would have insulation against the cold and plenty of fat reserves to burn through.)

Look, a couple of other things from the world of conventional dietetics bear looking at. Some experts disagree, but it has helped me understand the basic nature of food, and most particularly how your body breaks down the carbs into glucose – the basic fuel your body runs on – with your 'blood sugar' being the measure of how much glucose is in your blood. Some foods and some drinks break down quickly, some slowly. Things like cans of Coke quickly raise your blood sugar, as the glucose half of the sugar hits. It gives you a quick hit of energy, but in short order you are so hungry, you could 'eat the crotch out of a low flying duck', as the saying goes. Many dietitians characterise it as being like burning bunched-up paper in your fireplace. It will give you a quick burst of warmth, but once the flare has gone, the only way to get that warmth back is to keep feeding in more paper, keep drinking the Coke, keep eating the chocolate. Meantime, all the excess fructose in the Coke has been turned into fat, and has gone to your reserve tank!

Other foods, though, like boiled eggs and avocado, are slowly processed by your body. They slowly deliver nutrients, giving you precisely the slow burn you need, so *put another log on the fire, cook me up some bacon and some beans.*

Very broadly, natural foods, not yet broken down, burn long and strong, meaning you don't need constant top-ups. The main thing, Boomka, is that a working knowledge of all this is useful, as you generally need to put long-burning logs in your fire, not scrunched-up pieces of paper.

Here's the really simple version: It is not just obvious junk food that is bad for you, it's food that might not look like it's chock-a-block with calories, or foods that do a bloody great job at pretending they're healthy. More on this later!

And the real problem with junk food isn't just that it fills you up with calories that have no goodness attached, it's that it doesn't fill you up at all. You need more fast. Only an idiot, or someone trying to destroy their dodgy tax records, burns a fire with just paper. Be smart, stop burning paper as fuel, start burning logs. Junk food is junk, not just because Mum doesn't want you to have Coke and chips, but because it is JUNK. You are eating and drinking rubbish. Cut it out. Change your fuel, Boomka, and your gut will change back into a normal stomach.

And finally, one other thing to cover quickly is that all food has a level of fibre in it. It is that part of the food that cannot be broken down, and so inevitably must move through our digestive system. Generally speaking, the more fibre food has, the better our system works as the fibre takes the rest of the waste products with it, and our movements become more regular . . . but, moving right along!

(Unless, of course, you want to pursue the car analogy, in which case it's as if fibre makes your exhaust system work smoothly, allowing you to smoothly and regularly get rid of waste products.)

The main thing is that, ideally, this base level knowledge should equip you to understand what follows . . .

THREE

All the other solutions you've looked at (and what's wrong with them)

'In 2002, 231 million Europeans attempted some form of diet. Of these only 1 percent will achieve permanent weight loss.'
The New York Times

The scene was set at the 1999 cricket World Cup when Australia was playing Scotland at Worcester. Oh, go on, say you remember!

Late in the match, Scotland is going after the large Australian total, when your favourite and mine, Shane Warne, finds himself fielding way down in deep long-on, in front of a rowdy group of Scots, with a few Pommy blow-ins, who decided it would be a very good idea to pick on our Shane.

There are three reasons.

He is Shane Warne.

He is tabloid fodder from heaven for the British papers, with every day bringing new revelations about what he gets up to on Saturday nights. As the apocryphal yarn goes, a recent survey in *The Sun* had asked British women, 'Would you ever sleep with Shane Warne?' and no fewer than 72 per cent had replied, 'Never again!'

He is more than a tad on the portly side. To quote the late, great, P. G. Wodehouse in *Very Good, Jeeves*, he is 'a tubby little chap who looked as if he had been poured into his clothes and had forgotten to say "When!"'

But anyhoo, on this day, Warne is down there fielding the odd ball, and, of course, something of an organised choir of Scotsmen starts to form. Well practised, they break up into two sections of the choir, and on the cue of the choir leader dropping his raised arm, the first half sing out in a loud mock whisper:

Who ate all the pies?
Who ate all the pies?
Who ate all the pies?

The other section of the choir answer, singing in a crescendo:

Shane did!
Shane DID!
SHANE DID!!!!

And now altogether sing . . .

YOU FAT BASTARD, YOU FAT BASTARD, YOU ATE *ALL* THE PIES!

Warne being Warne, of course, simply shows them the finger but there is no doubt he is distinctly underwhelmed.

Now, whether or not this was the moment for the genesis of Shane Warne deciding, or at least his mum deciding, he needed to take diet pills, we know not – but we do know that that particular exercise ended in tears.

And doesn't it always?

Quite seriously, what kind of grown-ups believe in diet pills in the first place?

No, no, no, not you, Shane. *Grown-ups*, I said!

Ever since the Western world, particularly, started getting fat, from about the early 1980s onwards, there have been thousands, and I mean thousands, of solutions offered, and you and I – am I right, mate? – have tried more than our fair share, just as we've always had more than our fair share of food at the buffet!

The point is, most of the diets I discuss below fiddle around with the basic ratios of proteins/carbs/fats – while usually lowering the overall quantity. They lift or drop the protein or carbohydrate intake, according to the philosophy of the diet, and usually, but not always, reduce the level of fat. And hundreds of diets claim that simply by some magic combination of this food with that food, the weight will equally as magically fall off you. More often than not, one of these fad diets is promoted by one or many celebrities who embrace it, finally lose weight, and suddenly think they are nutritional experts. And if you think I am shifting uncomfortably at my own words, you are mistaken. First, I am not a celebrity, second, I don't claim to be an expert on nutrition at all – only to have a broad grasp of it – and finally what I will propose later in the book is not a diet at all. Rather, it is simply to understand what certain foods and drinks are doing to us, stop taking them, and let your body take care of the rest. But we will get to that.

In the meantime, most of those kind of magic diets are – to use the technical word – 'bullshit'.

Oh, come on. Look, if even *one* of them worked and could be easily sustained in the long term, everybody would be doing it. That there are so many of them is a fair sign that bugger-all of them work in the long run. In terms of promising big, and delivering nothing bar a brief feeling of virtue, they're just like religion – but don't get me started.

For let us cast our minds back to the dozens and dozens of failed fads of yore, the grapefruit diet, the Israeli Army diet, the Pritikin diet, the Pratkins diet (okay, I made that one up, but it would probably be just as effective as the others). What do they have in common? Everybody did them and then . . . they didn't. Because they didn't work. Or you couldn't keep following them, which meant they DIDN'T WORK. Let's look at some more popular failures, together with one or two that do have one or two redeeming features.

Herbal tea

The idea, of course, was that simply by drinking this tea, you could get slimmer. Seriously, mate? You tried that? How old are you? Can I get you interested then in selling you an Opera House and a Harbour Bridge? Going cheap! Of course slimming tea is complete and utter bullshit. Look, these slimming teas operate on exactly the same principle as any sort of 'superfood' like goji berries or kale or cacao. They aren't bad for you but nor are they going to make you lose weight. YOU are going to make you lose weight!

The best clue that it is dodgy?

Well, I reckon you can pick it by the fact that the last time I saw the most notorious promoter of slimming tea, Peter Foster, he still had a zebra suntan from the long time he spent in prison, and was crawling out from under the bushes, from whence the *Current Affair* crew had chased him. And yes, when he came out – without being nasty about it – it looked like he ate all the pies! Slim, he wasn't.

Okay, if you drink heaps of tea, at least you're not guzzling so many other drinks that do have calories, and you will lose weight if you stop drinking things that are bad for you (let's pause for a moment and all go 'DUH' together), but the notion that any tea can slim you down, in and of itself, is twaddle.

The 'fat melting' grapefruit diet

Lose five kilograms in 12 days!

Used with spectacular results by generations of celebrities! The grapefruit has a fat-burning enzyme, see . . .

See, there is rubbish, there is complete rubbish, and then there are diets which claim to boast a secret ingredient which allows you to get around the base level equation: you need to burn more calories than you are taking in. We might be dumb when it comes to food, Boomka, but we are not *this* dumb. Let us throw away our grapefruit, retain our dignity at least, and move on.

Xenical

This is as close as they have come to a pill that actually will take the weight off. The guts of the idea is that you can eat what you like, just as you ever have, but by popping a pill with every meal, you can line your gut with this thingammy, which would prevent you from digesting and absorbing fat into your bloodstream. I first heard about this over-the-counter drug in the late 1990s, and tried it shortly thereafter. The good thing? If I took it while having fatty food, I immediately felt a bit queasy, as if my body wasn't meant to take in that fat while I had those pills in me. The net result was that I tended to steer away from fatty foods.

The bad news? I am trying to think of a delicate way to put this. Those of you who have tried it will immediately know what I am talking about. What I am talking about is reminiscent of the time that Lord Nelson was on his flagship, *HMS Victory*, when the lookout shouts, 'Spanish ships on the port bow!'

In response, Nelson shouts for his cabin boy and says, 'Go to my cabin and bring me my three cornered hat, my sword and my red coat!'

A minute later, the boy comes back with the requested items and gives them to Nelson. As he hands them over he says to Nelson, 'I know why you want your hat and telescope, sir, but why do you want your red coat?'

'It's for camouflage,' Nelson replies. 'If I'm wounded in battle, the men will carry on fighting because they will be unable to see my blood because of the red coat that I wear, and because they'll not know that I'm injured, we may be able to defeat the Spanish.'

The Royal Navy, due to the forward thinking of Lord Nelson, sees off the Spanish.

A couple of days later the lookout shouts, 'Spanish fleet on the port bow.' Nelson brings his telescope to his one good eye and sees 500 Spanish ships, under full sail, coming straight for them!

In response, Nelson shouts for his cabin boy and says, 'Go to my cabin and bring me my three cornered hat, my sword, and my brown corduroy trousers.'

You get the drift.

Boomka, I am telling you, it is one of those things. If you haven't tried Xenical yet, my very simple suggestion is, *don't*. I am not going to go into details, and you can't make me, but the bottom line is if you're taking those pills, you simply cannot trust yourself to break wind. 'Cos the fat that doesn't go into your bloodstream has to go somewhere, and what happens is, the fat goes into your bowels, having not been processed and turned into energy. This results in a hideous, oily, sticky fluid of distinctly brown tinge. (Well – you did ask.) If you're lucky, it will emerge at the normal times, when you want it to. If you are *unlucky*, you will be at a black-tie dinner, about to get an award, hear your name called, and at that very moment, you will have to make the most excruciatingly uncomfortable walk of your life up to the podium. (Don't ask. Seriously, mate, *don't* ask.)

It's such an artificial solution, when the cause of the problem is entirely natural. Why go with Xenical when healthy eating, regular exercise and a little bit of self-control – say it after me, Boomka, 'self . . . *control* . . .' – will give a much better result (as well as keeping your pants and Reg Grundies clean)?

South Beach diet

Ten years ago, my brother Jim was one of many who read the bestselling book on this diet, took on the central concepts, and lost weight because of it. In essence, it relies on you eating 'slow-burning' foods with high fibre and lean protein. Carbs are divided up into good and bad. Good carbs are things like whole-wheat pasta and brown bread, while in the naughty corner are fruits, most vegetables, beans and legumes . . .

Phase One involves cutting down on fruits, most vegetables, beans and legumes. And you can't have any bread, rice, potatoes, pasta or baked goods. In their place you are supposed to eat a lot of proteins, good fats and 'non-starchy vegetables', whatever they are. (Seriously. Spare me formulaic diets where you feel like you need a science degree to understand them.)

In Phase Two, fruits, whole grains and vegetables are allowed back on the menu. You are also supposed to start exercising in this phase.

In Phase Three, you apparently know how to make good food decisions and you'll apparently be enthusiastic about your new healthy lifestyle.

The most telling detail of the book, the lightbulb moment for many, is what it says about processed foods.

Basically, to digest food, the body needs to break it down in six separate processes, and the South Beach diet maintains that generally, when you eat processed food, with modern white bread as a classic example, five of those six processes are already done. What that means is that when you have white bread, you can fill up very quickly, it goes down a treat, *and* get the energy surge – but only a short time afterwards, you are ravenous for more . . . and too often have it. It also advises steering away from any food that advertises 'Added fibre', or in fact Added anything, on the basis that it likely means they have nuked everything naturally occurring in the food and then put a bit of something back that is unnatural to it. Which is sensible.

And to be fair, if you stick to this plan, you will undeniably lose weight, as it is based on solid principles (more lean protein, fewer processed foods) and encourages exercise. The problem is that in the end it's just another diet. A few words of warning, however, are worth repeating. The British National Health Service report that some parts of the diet, which cut out carbs, cause side effects like 'tiredness, dizziness, insomnia, nausea and constipation'.

For me, it made my head hurt just trying to understand it all. It's like joining a cult and the Catholic Church at the same time: it's very complicated, there are a lot of restrictions and special rules, and you feel pious and guilty most of the time. I'm not saying it won't work for you, but why do so much work? Losing weight does not have to be this complicated because it will be unsustainable in the long run and when was the last time you heard of simple souls like us grasping complex diet plans, sticking to them, losing weight, and keeping it off?

Oh, and those of you who ever watched *Jamie's Kitchen* (unsurprisingly starring Jamie Oliver) will know another good reason to not try these type of diets. In the show, Oliver had just opened his swank new restaurant '13' in London, staffed by unemployed teens he had trained as staff and cooks. Oliver was informed that ex-President Bill Clinton would be coming to dine! Much frenzied food preparation takes place. Unfortunately, the ex-Prez has just gone on the South Beach diet. Cut to a fuming Jamie Oliver standing in the kitchen while a Clinton aide reads him a long list of dietary restrictions and explaining why all the dishes they have prepared are now unacceptable. Cut to Oliver in the carpark being pursued by the producer and camera crew as he leaves in a huff after explaining that he no longer wishes to meet or cook for the former President because it wasn't worth the bloody trouble and the next time he should bring his own bloody food to the restaurant or stay home.

Now, if this diet is too much trouble for Jamie Oliver, do you really think your and my cooking skills are up to it? Let us move on.

Atkins diet

Broadly, it works. But ... with a caveat or two. Ten years or so ago I ran into my mate, Adam Spencer, the brilliant mathematician from Sydney University, who turned into an even better speaker, writer and broadcaster. 'Cept this time I ran into him, he looked totally different – about

15 kilograms lighter than he had been only a couple of months earlier when I had last seen him.

As I would later find out from my own experience, when you have lost that much weight that quickly, there are only two possibilities: you are either very, very well. Or you are very, very unwell.

In Adam's case it was that he was very well. He had, he told me, embraced the Atkins/protein diet, which was built on a very scientific premise. If you give your body only protein, the body has to burn fat in your fat cells to get energy (your fat cells lose weight, mate, and so do you), and the weight just falls off you. Our reserve tank of fat that we talked about earlier inevitably gets smaller!

Adam maintained that, every meal, he had as much bacon, eggs and sausages as he liked, but just had no bread, pasta, rice or anything that was not solid protein. The two riders he added was that he had to have heaps of water with it, to wash it all through, and he wouldn't recommend staying on it for more than two weeks at a time, as your body couldn't cope.

I tried it. I totally focused on doing *exactly* as he said – 'cept I didn't pile it on my plate – for about two weeks, which was as long as I could stand in any case. I did not have a single carb. And the weight did indeed *fall off*. To my stunned amazement, every day I was taking off between quarter and half a kilo and by the end of it, I had dropped five kilos in a fortnight.

There were two problems. For those two weeks, I just didn't feel right. I always felt full, with that same really uncomfortable feeling you get when you haven't been to the loo for a while . . . for the very good reason that I hadn't.

I also had low energy, a sort of buzz in my head that wouldn't go away, and cramps. I couldn't think straight for craving something, anything, that wasn't protein. As to bad breath, I'm telling you, I could curl your hair from a distance of five metres.

And second, once I reverted to my usual eating pattern, the weight all came back nearly as quickly. (I kid you not, one of the most aggravating things I found on this journey to health has been to discover that most of the wankers who used to carry on about it 30 years ago were absolutely right, and I was absolutely wrong. And they have always been healthy and svelte, while I have been an oft' unhealthy – what's that expression again? – 'Fatty Boomka'.)

Despite all that, when I was religiously following Atkins, it was the best thing for rapid weight loss I've ever come across. I also note that people like Kim Kardashian endorse it but, despite that, I am told by the experts Atkins is still the most rational diet metabolically speaking, as long as you're not on it forever. Still, I also can't help but note that, just as Jim Fixx, the bloke credited with popularising jogging as a mass pastime, died with his running shoes on, just after jogging, at the age of only 52, so too is it endlessly repeated – because it is simply too good not to – that Atkins himself carked it with sclerotic arteries, caked with so much congealed fat that the blood couldn't get through. In fact, it was nothing of the sort! He died of an 'epidural hematoma' – that was a lecture I missed when *not* attending Med School – but I am advised it had nothing to do with his diet.

As critics point out, however, that does not change the fact that the Atkins diet is about as far from balanced as you can get – and I am advised there are some health risks if you stay on it long term, most particularly if you have kidney problems.

Plus you won't stay on it, mate. I didn't and very few do. Yes, Adam bloody Spencer did – dipping into and out of it when he needs to lose weight – but he is extra special, isn't he? He is what we call an 'outlier', or more simply he is not typical. I know your weaknesses, mate, because I share them, and while solemnly agreeing to only eat bacon and sausages sounds like a brilliant scam, we both know what is going to happen. You will be back to bread. And pasta. And pastry.

Isn't there a better way? Yes. Read on.

Stomach stapling

One of my closest friends who will remain nameless – let's just call him Joe Hockey – had it done. Joe has always been a big man. My long-time claim has been that when I die, Joe will be one of the eight men to carry my coffin, while, if he dies first, I will be one of the 24 poor bastards carrying his . . .

But I digress.

On a Monday morning three years ago, I pleaded with the then Federal Treasurer not to go to the hospital – where I knew he was about to have two-thirds of his stomach removed – on the grounds that it was akin to self-mutilation. Joe, as he was ever wont to do in the face of my advice, ignored me and went ahead.

The result? It worked, sort of. That is, though he was knocked around a bit by the surgery, he did indeed go on to lose heaps of weight – about 30 kilos – upon the simple reckoning that these days he simply can't heartily tuck into a three-course meal even if he wanted to. (This is more than useful in his current role as our man in Washington, as part of his full-on and flat-out job is to live in a house with six staff – the Embassy must constantly entertain dignitaries – and it means His Excellency cannot spit over his shoulder without hitting one of his staff in the eye as she is offering a cream bun.)

Other versions of the same surgery are things like **Vertical Banded Gastroplasty Surgery**, which is every bit as nasty as it sounds. They open your tummy, and slip a band and metal staples around the top part of the stomach, to create a small pouch with a one-centimetre opening to the rest of the stomach. Same principle as above, it's just that, like the stomach stapling, it's expensive, painful and has *shockin'* side effects if you don't eat slowly. (The least of these is vomiting up partially digested food.) And you have trouble eating enough of the right foods to get proper nutrition. Can there ever be a more unnatural and extreme solution to what is a natural problem?

Many, too – not the redoubtable Joe – complain about a loss of energy. That is, their body is designed to have a certain sized fuel tank to call on. When, through whatever method, you restrict the size of that fuel tank, it stands to reason, yes, that you will frequently run out of gas.

Also, these guys are cheating. They didn't lose weight, the surgeon lost it for them. And it's unnecessary surgery, which as Joan Rivers is no longer able to tell you, is not a good idea. Don't go under the knife, Fatty, *change* your life. Safer, simpler, better.

The weird sex diet

A very good mate of mine, very well known to me – exactly my weight, age and background – was briefly put on the weird sex diet by his wife, the basic idea being that if he achieves his target weight, they get to have weird sex. And if he gets five kilos below that weight, next time *he* gets to wear the nurse's outfit!

It worked. For a while.

Jenny Craig

You know the drill. Look, if you follow it to the letter, it more or less works – at least while you're on it. How can it *not* work? I went on it for about two months back in the late 1990s and did indeed drop about six kilos. But there are a couple of downsides, the first and most obvious one of which is that you need to pay through the nose! You're coughing up roughly 18 dollars a day to have some-one else cook and deliver food to your door. In theory, that's a great system. It's like never ending room service, and who doesn't want that? Have someone else do the hard work for you AND lose weight?! You bloody beauty. But for a penetrating glimpse into the bleeding bloody obvious, what happens when you go off Jenny Craig? You're back where you started, Boomka – getting fatter every day. Jenny Craig is a temporary and expensive fix to a long-term problem. *Much* better to address the real problem and get on top of it, forever, than stuff around with expensive temporary solutions like JC.

Plus plenty of blokes find they are paying money for food they don't really enjoy. That's like formally agreeing to go to a bad restaurant where you are not enjoying yourself every day for a year. Would a sane person do this? You are not a baby, Boomka, cook for yourself, just cook the right things. There. Saved you $540 a month. You're welcome.

The 5:2 diet

The basis of the 5:2 diet is five days of 'unmoderated' eating, and then fasting for the other two. On the fasting days you are allowed to have scrambled eggs for breakfast and perhaps some tea or coffee, and a few nibbles during the rest of the day – but you must keep your intake to no more than 600 calories on fasting days. Women should limit themselves to 500 calories. The broad philosophy is that this is what it was like for cavemen and women, who would hunt their game, feast on it, and then hunt again. (After all, Raquel Welch *did* look pretty amazing in *One Million Years B.C.*) The 5:2 diet achieved popularity from celebrity endorsement and bestselling books in the UK and US, but the British National Health Service deems it an ineffective fad diet. Critics of the diet maintain the fasting alone is likely to result in difficulties sleeping, bad breath, anxiety, severe dehydration and unexplained periods of exhaustion. And they also note that while fasting can be quite good for you, the other major problem with this diet is that if you spend those five days drinking alcohol, smashing donuts and going to the drive-through at Mickey D's, you may develop kidney and liver problems in the long term. No amount of fasting is going to solve that, much less two days every week.

To be fair, some people *do* swear by the 5:2 diet, and they seem to me to be the ones who don't actually blow out on those five days. A mate of mine from Sydney University lost 14 kilograms fairly quickly three years ago, and has kept it off, simply by pursuing 5:2. On the strength of his success, I read the book, tried it and indeed dropped a couple of kilos over as many weeks. In my experience, however, on the days I was fasting I just couldn't get my brain into gear. It felt like I was trying to start the engine with no fuel in the tank. Meantime, I kid you not, my friend 'Pizza' saw a story on *60 Minutes* about the new wonder diet on a Sunday night, started it on Monday morning but was so ravenous by 10 am that day he had a packet of Tim Tams.

This is you, Boomka. This is me. In the end we are all 'Pizza'. Accept it and wave farewell to another fair-weather fad.

Counting every calorie, in and out

A good friend of mine, Fairfax economics writer Jessica Irvine, brought out a book called *The Bottom Line* a couple of years ago, with an interesting premise. Broadly: your body is like an economy.

'Weight loss comes down not to fad diets,' she explained, 'but to one very simple equation: calories in minus calories out. It's accounting – just like the federal budget, with its incoming revenue and outgoing expenses. But unlike the federal budget, deficits are the order of the day when it comes to weight loss.'

Now, to lose a full kilogram of fat, the deficit must reach 7700 calories, ideally by small steady decrements. If, say, you spent Monday through to Sunday in a caloric deficit of 1100 every day, by the end of the week you would have reached the 7700 calories and lost the kilo. Maintain that daily deficit for two weeks, and you'd be two kilos lighter. And so on and so forth. Helped by calorieking.com.au, she set out to measure her calorie intake, as precisely as she did how many calories she burned through exercise, by wearing a heart rate monitor.

It revealed to her that while there are more calories in a large fries at McDonald's – 453 of the brutes – than in an entire healthy dinner, there are just 63 calories in an entire punnet of strawberries. So eat the strawberries instead! And she got her head around the unequal relationship between intake and exercise, to the effect that, 'It takes less than a minute to devour a burger with 600 calories, but two hours of brisk walking to burn it off.'

In sum?

'The body needs energy to fuel whatever movement you do,' she explained. 'It has two main sources: what you put in your mouth or the fat sitting in your fat cells. Deny it enough of the first source, and the body will dig into the second. Hey presto, bye bye bottom.'

Speaking of which . . .

'The bottom line is our bottom lines have been crying out for a good accountant. We must take back control of our own bodies.'

Bravo. Jess and I were sort of on the same track at the same time, and the point of her journey was that going through all that malarkey of counting everything changed the way she lived and she has kept it off since.

Which is fabulous for her. And the approach clearly works – for her. But you and me, mate? Frankly, I would sooner put hot knitting needles in my eyes than tabulate so precisely the calorific intake of everything I eat, putting it on a spreadsheet, working out how much I burn, etc. The principle is fine, and it's useful to know that the average Australian male burns around 2200 calories a day, and that with just one Ultimate Double Whopper from Hungry Jack's (1141 calories), or a Double Quarter Pounder from McDonald's (853 calories), you've just about blown half the bank right there. And we also need to know such rough yardsticks as that briskly walking the dog for an hour is estimated to burn about 300 calories, while if you dance for the same period it goes up to 400 calories; cycling moderately fast = 480 calories; doing lap after lap of breast-stroke = 860 calories; while if you're crazy enough to box for 60 minutes it goes up to over 1000 calories, etc.

But accurately measuring it all?

I reckon for you and me, Boomka, it would be murder on a stick. I want to work out the broad brushstrokes of the eating and exercise plan I live by, the central values, and take it from there, while still being obsessive about a few key things, but we will get to that. Calorie counting is not for us! I hate to say it, son, but I think religiously following all the rules and regulations that come with such a plan is perilously close to that worst of all possible things: Un-Australian.

At the very least, un-Australian-male! And, yes, I do mean that, by the way. As a species, we have *never* been at our best following precise orders. This much was documented by an English officer, Major-General Hubert Essame, after closely observing the way our own General John Monash – more on him later – was able to get our Diggers to achieve such magnificent results in the final months of 1918, as the Great War neared its end:

> 'As an Australian, [Monash] realised that he must appeal to [the Diggers'] intelligence, their imagination, their adaptability, their high sense of comradeship, their capacity for independent judgement and their aggressive instincts. He would feed them on victory. He would teach them to believe, because of success, that they were invincible. He would make every man feel that what he was and what he did was vital.'

See, the Diggers could never just blindly follow orders. It wasn't in them. But give them a goal, and the reasons why taking that goal was important, and they were the best of the best, and when in France, *la crème de la crème*!

Move on.

The Malcolm Turnbull diet

A year or so before he became PM, I ran into Malcolm Turnbull at a Perth hotel, and was stunned at how much he'd lost since the last time I'd seen him a couple of months earlier – making him probably two stone lighter than he was when Chair of the Australian Republican Movement, where I'd first got to know him. I asked his secret.

He told me he got there by not eating . . . until he felt as though he would faint. Then, and only then, would he munch on a vegetable or have a concoction put together by a Chinese herbalist, Dr Shuquan Liu, who runs a practice in Turnbull's electorate.

'The way to lose weight is to eat less,' Malcolm told the press, 'so I ate a lot less for a month and lost a lot of weight pretty quickly.'

And he does mean a *lot* less.

'I must say that I found the fast extremely informative,' Turnbull said, 'because it made me realise I am in control of my own body and can control my appetite. It is a very good insight.'

Malcolm later went on to lose 93 kilos of extraneous weight from the cabinet in a single day by knifing my old rugby coach, Tony Abbott.

I'm joking! Tony is 87 kilos at worst. Okay, the diet worked for him, but that's Malcolm Turnbull, with a drive and discipline that could scare a Great White Shark. You and I aren't made like that.

The Paleo diet

This one is a biggie. The idea behind this diet is that we should eat only the kind of food our ancestors ate. This is a very serious diet based on the sound idea of eating the same kind of food that made our ancient ancestors short, primitive and have a life expectancy of about as many winters as there were days between full moons. So, obviously, no processed food for starters, but also no wheat, dairy, vegetable oil, grains, sugar, legumes or preservatives. But you can have plant foods, nuts, berries, grass-fed meat, herbs and spices – as long as they are not part of the 11 secret herbs and spices on KFC – and you can also rip into fermented drinks such as kefir, whatever that is, and coconut water. I have never tried it, and frankly don't know anyone who has, but it has been pilloried in the press as little more than last year's fad, suggesting that while there is heavyweight marketing behind it, and lots of products like paleo brownies, paleo bread and cookies, as Dr Joanna McMillan noted, our paleo parents 'did not have brownies even if they are made of raw cacao, avocado and coconut oil'.[1]

Skip it, Skipper.

CSIRO diet

Like Atkins, this is another of those rarest of popular diets that is actually based on serious science! The foundation stone is eating lots of lean meat and *heaps* of vegies, a diet developed by the mighty CSIRO back in 2005. Mostly it is common sense. Anything with high protein and low carbs works, if being a little dull. Look, I don't know if you've ever met someone from the CSIRO but they are not exactly Hunter S. Thompson meets Keith Richards. They are dry, sensible, earnest and dull. Can it be a coincidence that these are also the food groups they enjoy? You be the judge. But to be fair to the CSIRO, this one seems to be regarded by the serious boffins, and in my own experience, as far and away the best of the lot. Based on science, it broadly works, because it knocks the sugar out of your intake.

At the end of the day, however, it is still a diet. And what we need with you, mate, is to get your head out of the whole notion of 'going on a diet', which inevitably means you will 'go off the diet'.

No, mate, we need you to *evolve* your whole mind-set. None of the solutions outlined so far are the answer, because even at best they are short-term solutions to what is a long-term problem. They don't get close to the heart of the issue, they just undo some of the damage done, for a short time, before you go back to business as usual, and the problem gets worse.

So, here's the thing, the first basic concept it took me 30 years of adult life to get my head around:

*The thing is not to go on a diet, it is simply to **change** your diet.*

FOUR

Giving up sugar

'Once you're sensitised to negative effects of unhealthy choices, it gets easier to turn down what used to seem impossible to resist . . .'
Mark Sisson, author of The Primal Diet
Translated, he's saying once you understand the crap that is in crap food, and how it roots your whole system, you no longer want it.

'I was eating three pieces of fruit a day, a handful of dried fruit, a teaspoon or two of honey in my tea, a small (35g) bar of dark chocolate after lunch and, after dinner, honey drizzled on yoghurt, or dessert (if I was out). A conservative day would see me consume about 25-plus teaspoons of sugar, just in that rundown of snacks above. That's not counting the hidden sugar in things like tomato sauce and commercial breads. I told myself I ate 'good' sugar and convinced myself I didn't have a problem.'
Damon Gameau in That Sugar Film

So what *is* the solution to this whole weight-loss caper?

I thought you'd never ask.

After having already taken, as discussed, a Dennis Lillee run-up to this, I am sure you won't mind if I lope in for another couple of steps.

So there I was, on a family holiday in Africa in early 2012. All five of us were standing upon the bridge that goes over the Zambezi River, just down from Victoria Falls, about to do a bungee jump.

There were two key problems. The first was that one of the family members was something close to a shuddering wreck at the mere *contemplation* of jumping, let alone actually doing it. The second was that the pathetic, and I use the word advisedly, family member in question was . . . *me*.

A little over 90 minutes later . . . cometh the crunch time.

Ahead of me, just two steps more . . . the abyss.

Behind me, my wife and three teenage children, all of whom had jumped with joy, were now watching me closely.

No joke, this was as serious as syphilis. Just the week before, a young Australian woman had jumped from this very spot, only to have the rope break. She had mercifully survived, but still. That was the reason they'd stopped the pure bungee thing, and now, if I jumped, I would fall about 80 metres before going out on a kind of swing. Eighty freaking metres! Two steps ahead . . . the gaping maw of my own mortality beckoned. Two steps back . . . humiliation.

I jumped . . . (*Actually, if it please the court, Your Honour, I was pushed! I kid you not, the Zambian blokes behind me*

*got tired of all my carry-on. They made sure I was secure, and
gave me a bump.*)

COMMMMME . . . . TO . . . . JESUS!

People who bungee often report a staggeringly euphoric,
liberating feeling as they fall – including my wife, and all
three kids. Which is fabulous for them. The ones who have
the rope break on them are seldom available for comment . . .

I, however, hated it. Every single wretched second of it.
Never again. The only good thing about it was getting to
grasp the bridge again about ten minutes later, after they –
and they gathered half the nearby village, *'Come quick, come
quick, and bring the elephants, we need help!'* – had hauled
me up again.

The worst of it, though, after asking Lisa very quietly
if she could retrieve the brown trousers from my bag, was
being told I had set a post-war record for the heaviest bloke
to have jumped. Seriously? A place frequented by American
tourists, blokes who never saw hamburgers they didn't
want to throw down their throats like Fantales, who regard
guzzling Coke as the second-most important human right
after the right to buy AK-47s from their local supermarket,
and *I* was the heaviest?

Quel embarrassment!

I mean, I knew that before jumping I had jumped on
their scales, and they had registered 146 kilograms, but
I had taken that in the same magnanimous spirit in which I
took African hot-water taps sometimes gushing cold water,
their electric light system being a little on the intermittent
side of things, and their people frequently mistaking me for

Hulk Hogan. I love Africa and its people, but not everything works the way it does in Kansas, Dorothy; and while I was amused that their scales could be so far out of whack, I hadn't taken it seriously. But *now*, as I lay, post-jump, exhausted, they were all agreeing *I* was the heaviest! And, I must say, the photos Lisa took *did* make me look a tad on the cuddly side of things.

It made me more determined than ever to finish reading the book I had brought with me on the holiday, David Gillespie's *Sweet Poison*. Gillespie, a Brisbane lawyer by trade, had struggled with his weight for years and tried many of the diets and solutions I mentioned in the previous chapter. His own 'Come to Jesus' moment was when his wife told him that she was pregnant with twins, meaning they would soon have six kids, when he was flat out coping, and *fat* out hoping to find the energy for just four kids. So he began researching, trying to get to the absolute bottom of why he was hungry all the time, and had blown out a massive 40 kilograms from what his weight should have been. Most impressively, he delved beyond the standard answer of 'you're eating too much', and didn't accept that because people were experts in various fields they were necessarily right. He found the answer, published it, and his book *Sweet Poison* was the result.

Sure, there was a bit of scientific mumbo jumbo in there that I didn't necessarily get – taking food content down to its molecular level – but the premise was dead simple: sugar is killing us all. (Not just because it is making us fat, either. He makes many other credible claims, most particularly warming to a theme that links sugar to various kinds of cancer, but that part is beyond the ken of this book.)

From a dietary point of view, the crux of the problem is not just the calories those sugary foods and drinks add, but how *hungry* it makes you for more sugary things and everything else besides; how, after the first Tim Tam, you're immediately hungry for a second and third, not to mention – after that delightful afternoon snack – a much bigger dinner.

The whole problem starts with the shocking difference between how much sugar our bodies are designed to cope with and how much we *actually* take in.

The latter figure should stun you.

Though the figures are wildly disputed and there is no definitive data, Gillespie's credible calculations are that the average Australian and American consumes at least 36 teaspoons of sugar a day, which, at four grams a teaspoon, adds up to about a kilo of sugar a week, which translates into over 50 freaking kilograms a year! (And that's the *average*, mate. So what must it have been for you and me? When was the last time you and I did *average* consumption of food and drink?)

This is all the more shocking when you realise the natural intake of our ancestors – the amount our body actually hums on best, if not actually needs – was about two kilograms a year, or, in their case, the weight of two mid-sized rocks.

Savvy, mate?

Focus! Because this is the guts of it. You'll excuse me if I get a tad repetitive. We've inherited from our ancestors a beautifully efficient human machine, designed to run on a certain kind of natural fuel. And a key part of that natural fuel, for our motor to run sweetly, is that – as evidenced by the levels of consumption pre-industrialisation – it only takes in as many teaspoons of sugar a day as you used to put in your coffee. That is, just over a teaspoon a day, and for the record, our body can get by fine without any at all. But when we guzzle just one can of Coca-Cola, we are taking in about 39 grams of sugar, as in well over NINE teaspoons! You get it?

With just one can of Coke we are taking in our *entire* weekly ration! Every bit of sugar beyond that which is surplus, more or less has to finish up as extra weight.

Keep guzzling Cokes, on top of a diet that delivers enough calories already, and of course you will turn into the Michelin Man. How else could it work?

One of the most internationally accomplished researchers in the world on the subject of sugar, Professor Alejandro Gugliucci, with whom I have extensively consulted, said to me, 'Some humans had access to ripening fruit, very occasionally, and usually no more than once a year. We did not evolve to get a sudden hit of 40 grams of fructose in liquid form, with no food – like kids do with two or three cans of soda – at all. It ruins our human machine, perfected over a million years.'

Remember what I said earlier about the stomach being your fuel tank, and the flab around your belly and elsewhere being the rubbery reserve tank, this huge malleable bladder that expands when filled with fat? When we put that much sugar through our system, there can be only one result. We get a reserve tank ten times, and worse, the size of the original fuel tank.

Compounding the problem is that while too much sugar blows out our reserve tank, so too does it completely root our fuel gauge – the thing in our body that tells us when we are full. See, the gauge only works if we put in natural fuel, and is completely buggered when we overload it with food that has a completely unnatural concentration of sugar.

Look, I'll expand on all this below, but for now that's the way to think of it, and I repeat, if you only get one thing from this book, get this: **stop the sugar = stop the hunger**. If somebody had drummed that into my noggin 25 years ago, I would never have even got close to 152 kilograms.

But once you get it, and embrace it, everything starts to come good. For some blokes, the weight just melts away slowly. For me, once I cut the sugar, I was very quickly on the road to a massive slim-down and the weight just flew off. Stop the sugar and stop the hunger was the blinding breakthrough that led me to drop 42 kilograms so far – certainly not without effort, but crucially without gnawing hunger pangs, and without having to think about it all the damn time.

Stop the sugar, and your body tells you when you've had enough food.

Stop the sugar, and your fuel gauge – which has likely been on the blink for 30 or 40 years – starts to work and tells you when to stop eating and drinking.

Stop the sugar, and together with the fuel gauge, so too does the right blinker and accelerator start to work! Listen as your engine starts to purr again. You can finally take the hand-brake off, throw it into gear and at last pull out onto the road once more as you are soon moving out after the pack again.

Stop the sugar, and before your very eyes, you turn into the bloke who pushes the plate away and says to the hostess, 'Thank you, Martha, but I couldn't *possibly* have any more of that mashed potato, as I find I am *teddibly, teddibly* full,' and you'll mean it!

At the time of reading Gillespie's book and embarking on the new way of eating, I was doing some work for the Channel Seven *Sunday Night* program. When the executive producer, Mark Llewellyn, noticed the beginnings of my fairly sudden weight loss, they were quick to get the cameras on me, playing touch football and basketball, and running along the beach with my top off, so they could record the last of my days as a still fairly fat man, before following my journey downwards. (To see the story, google 'FitzSimons, *Sweet Poison, Sunday Night*'.)

Over the course of that program, I went down from just above 140 kilograms, all the way to 122 kilograms, and was able to interview the most renowned expert in the world on the dangers of sugar, Dr Robert Lustig, of San Francisco, and a whole new world opened up to me.

For, as I discovered, David Gillespie was *not* a lone, loony maverick, as some portray him, but simply part of a growing movement for sanity that has been slowly gathering momentum for decades. Lustig is currently at the forefront of it, and the aforementioned Professor Alejandro Gugliucci is one of his closest associates. After a slow start, work in the field is surging forward around the world.

An article in the *Guardian* called 'The Sugar Conspiracy', by the esteemed English journalist Ian Leslie, sets out the historical background superbly. With a little of my own research added to flesh out the detail that interests me, it goes something like this . . .

Back on 23 September 1955, the President of the United States, Dwight D. Eisenhower, was taking a few days to visit his in-laws, where he took the opportunity, between puffing on his ubiquitous cigarettes, to play golf at the Cherry Hills Country Club.

About to tee off on the eighth hole, he began suffering what felt like a sudden burst of indigestion. Alas, over the next 12 hours, this turned into serious chest pains. As it turned out, of course, it was not indigestion at all, but rather that thing that had been relatively uncommon in America before the Second World War, but was becoming distressingly more frequent in this era: 'a heart attack'.

The following day, Dr Paul Dudley White, the leading cardiologist in the land – who, after losing his sister to rheumatic heart disease at a young age had devoted his life to studying the heart thereafter – fronted a packed press conference, where he gave fair warning to all how they could avoid the same fate as the President.

Steer away from foods laden with fat, as that would lift your cholesterol, which would in turn risk clogging your arteries. White was quick to cite the work of a nutritionist and epidemiologist at the University of Minnesota, Ancel Keys, who was convinced that the culprit behind most heart attacks was consuming an excess of saturated fats, through eating too much fatty food like cheese, bacon, red meat, butter and so forth. After all, wasn't that common sense?

To begin with, it was backed up by the English language itself: overweight people are called 'fat', the same word as Keys identified as the prime culprit in food they ate – fat – to make them that way. Plus, it made sense after base-level scientific analysis, given that one gram of fat contained twice as many calories as a gram of protein or carbohydrate.

Further, a brilliant, forceful man, Keys had many influential adherents in the medical establishment, and his notion that fat in the food caused fat in the arteries quickly became the orthodoxy. Just as the notion that an anvil would fall to earth much faster than a nail was also once the orthodoxy – because it just made sense.

The leading nutritionist in Great Britain, John Yudkin, however, became convinced that the real problem was not fat at all, but excessive consumption of sugar – the fructose half of which is processed in the liver, turns to fat and then enters the bloodstream. After all, he noted, mankind had been eating meat since the dawn of time and it had only been in recent decades that sugar – 'a pure carbohydrate, with all fibre and nutrition stripped out' – had become a significant part of that diet as well. Could it be coincidence that once-rare heart attacks were now suddenly showing up as a frequent occurrence at the same time as this sudden prevalence of sugar?

'To Yudkin's thinking,' Leslie recounted, 'it seemed more likely to be the recent innovation, rather than the prehistoric staple, making us sick.'

Yudkin's first published foray into the field, noting the dangers of sugar, came in 1957, placing him as a direct opponent, across the Atlantic, to Keys.

Still, Yudkin's ideas were initially well received. Gathering his ideas, and continuing his research, he put them all in a book released in 1972, called *Pure, White, and Deadly*, where he was scathing about sugar.

'If only a small fraction of what we know about the effects of sugar were to be revealed in relation to any other material used as a food additive,' he wrote, 'that material would promptly be banned.'

And so the battle lines were set for the clash that goes on to this day.

What Keys and his adherents had, and still have, on their side is the aforementioned common sense: it simply stands to reason that too much fatty pork on your fork should be the source of the problem of fat clogging up your veins. Ditto, too much butter on your toast. Double ditto, dripping fat from your chops. And, of course, Keys was fully supported by the ever more powerful industry that had grown wealthy by selling food products packed with sugar.

Among those who soon came to attack Yudkin's claims were scientists from both the British Sugar Bureau and the World Sugar Research Organisation – the first a lobby group for the sugar industry, the second an international scientific body funded by the same. And there was a lot of it about. Even as this book is going to press, a major story has broken in the US about how, back in the 1960s, heavyweight Harvard nutritionists 'published two reviews in a top medical journal downplaying the role of sugar in coronary heart disease. Newly unearthed documents reveal what they didn't say: A sugar industry trade group initiated and paid for the studies, examined drafts, and laid out a clear objective to protect sugar's reputation in the public eye.'

Marion Nestle, one of the world's most famous nutrition experts, from New York University, was appropriately scathing: 'Science is not supposed to work this way. Is it really true that food companies deliberately set out to manipulate research in their favor? Yes, it is, and the practice continues."[1]

Beyond such corruption, however, how could honest and uncorrupted scientists not only come to such opposing conclusions, but stand by them for decades? One reason, as I have discovered in the course of writing and researching this book, is that nutritional science is evolving quickly, and is a world heavy on complex theories rather than incontrovertible facts accepted by all. And even facts that are widely accepted can lead to startlingly different conclusions. Only slowly is the battle being won as ever more research is conducted, and yes, as ever more people like me, point to staggering and sustained weight loss and improved health, simply by embracing one of the theories.

#IstandwithYudkin #Ilost40KgswithLustig

The bottom line of the struggle between the theories of Keys and Yudkin is that over the coming years, Yudkin and his crazy idea, that too much sugar was the prime culprit in causing too much fat and subsequent heart conditions – as opposed to Keys' bleeding obvious and common-sense contention that it was too much fat in the food causing too much fat in the arteries – were completely discredited.

No matter that Yudkin's extensive studies and accumulated data supported exactly this, while Keys' own data simply didn't fit his narrative. Yudkin was howled down, harassed high and hit low.

'Can you wonder,' he noted mournfully before he died, in 1995, 'that one sometimes becomes quite despondent about whether it is worthwhile trying to do scientific research in matters of health?'

Vindication for his ideas would not arrive for decades, and even now – as I write in 2016 – the battle is far from won.

But they're getting there . . .

FIVE

A little science, anyone?

'A *Weight Loss* book written by Physicists would be
1 sentence long: "Consume calories at a lower rate than
your body burns them".'
Neil deGrasse Tyson, famous American physicist

As scientific research and data-sharing became ever more
globalised, Yudkin's case really did become ever more supported. Bolshie boffins started to mow down what seemed to
be common sense and instead supported the Englishman's
original seemingly counterintuitive conclusions.

Leslie notes, 'France, the country with the highest intake of
saturated fat, has the lowest rate of heart disease; Ukraine, the
country with the lowest intake of saturated fat, has the highest.'

Tribal societies such as the Inuits and Massai, which live
on traditional, nearly all-fat diets, have practically no record
of heart disease at all.

In America, scientific pioneers like Dr Robert Lustig pushed ahead on their own research, and came to their own independent conclusions.

Visiting Adelaide in 2008 to speak at a conference, Dr Lustig was approached after his talk by an Australian scientist who asked whether he had read Yudkin, who had been beating Lustig's drum four decades earlier.

Lustig shook his head but was careful to dig out a copy of the book when he got back to the States . . . and was stunned.

'Holy crap,' Lustig recounted his feelings. 'This guy got there 35 years before me.'

If you really want to get into the science behind his views then put Lustig and *Sugar: The Bitter Truth* through your search engine and watch his seminal 2009 lecture, which goes for 90 minutes. In it, Lustig calls fructose nothing less than a 'poison', all but singularly culpable for America's epidemic of obesity.

When I interviewed Lustig, it was quickly clear just how serious he was. The Californian is so convinced of the damage that sugar does that he maintains that the likes of Coke and all such sugary soft drinks should not be sold to those under 18. When I asked him if he would prefer a 15-year-old have a wine or a Coke, he insisted the wine would be less damaging.

On that general subject of the damage done by consuming alcohol versus sugar, he is firm on the ground that a far bigger problem than Americans suffering from beer belly is what he calls . . . well, you tell 'em, Doc . . . 'soda belly, that's what America is suffering from – no ifs, ands or buts, that's what it is'.

And it makes sense, does it not? Drinking just one can of Coke a day, you're putting over nine teaspoons of extra sugar through your system, and an extra 160 calories. That is $365 \times 150 = 58,400$ calories, per year. Now they reckon that for every 7700 calories you don't burn, you gain a kilogram of fat. That means that over the year, just one can of Coke, alone, is adding over seven and a half kilograms a year of fat that you must burn through! And if you don't, it stays. A freaking STONE in the old money! And that's just the Coke alone, before you count the extra crap you're eating because it makes you so hungry. Mate, I can't put it any simpler, you have to stop drinking that shit, and the same goes for fruit juices. It is sheer madness. You will recall how you and I used to love smoking, but are now disgusted by it. You need to get to the same point with soft drink and fruit juice. I have.

Now, while Dr Lustig is at the scientific prow of the global anti-sugar movement, the British chef Jamie Oliver – who I also interviewed for Channel Seven – is the global celebrity face of it, trying to make the world see sense on sugar. His greatest stunt, as you might see in the piece I did for *Sunday Night*, was shocking a group of American parents with how much sugar was going down the gullets of their kids through flavoured milk alone: 57 tonnes of it, which filled a Los Angeles school bus just behind him. And cut! The shocked look on their faces said it all.

And of course in recent years there have also been a slew of documentaries exposing the underbelly of the whole food industry when it comes to whacking sugar into everything.

The thrust of Gillespie is entirely consistent with all of the above.

From first to last he maintained that if you just cut sugar from what you are eating and drinking, then everything else would come good.

Now, to be unfair, a lot of dietitians who I have talked to about Gillespie sneer unpleasantly and insist on pointing out – thank you, I know – that this bloke is a Brissie lawyer, not a trained dietitian, but I don't care.

As illustrated above, he is not some whacko from Waco, proclaiming untested nonsense. Rather, his stuff is simply the latest burst of sanity in a debate that has been going for 50 years. And, most importantly for me, he put it in language that even a rugby second-rower could understand, telling me something I didn't know.

I read Gillespie's stuff, embraced it – modified his approach on a couple of things that particularly suit me and my lifestyle, which I will expand on below – consulted widely with others in the same anti-sugar movement, and lost something nudging towards a third of my body weight.

His entire book, *Sweet Poison*, is really worth reading – particularly if you want a more scientific explanation of what I have offered above – and I highly recommend it, and all the more so because David has become a friend and been so generous in helping me with these chapters of the book.

The key concern of the anti-sugar brigade is that everyone understands what they have learned, that the absolute key for most of us to get back to better health is to cut back our sugar intake to what it was always meant to be: three-fifths – you should actually carefully measure it out – of bugger-all. In fact, Lustig made the point to my 'best bud', American actor Alec Baldwin – more on him later – that there is no damage done if you do get to bugger-all.

'There is not one biochemical reaction in your body, not one, that requires dietary fructose, not one that requires sugar. Dietary sugar is completely irrelevant to life. People say, oh, you need sugar to live. Garbage.'

So let's get to an understanding of what happens when we do take sugar into our system, and look at the very basic background science behind it. Time to think back on how it was before the industrialisation of food production came along.

See, back in prehistoric days, sweetness served a very useful evolutionary purpose.

Me, Urg.

Me, live in cave.

Me, not sure if this plant good or bad to eat.

Me, taste.

If sweet, me eat. If bitter, me spit out as either poison or maybe a donkeysaurus pissed on it just before I got here.

Get it?

We are designed to like sweetness as a signal that particular plant life is good to eat and a likely source of high energy, or even, as in the case of maturing fruit, letting us know it's ready to eat. As one who grew up on an orange orchard, I know better than most that a Valencia orange picked too soon can be as bitter as a Wallaby loss to England. But just a few months later, the same fruit can be as sweet as the first ball of an Ashes campaign taking an English wicket.

The point is, the sweeter it is, the more likely it is to provide the energy we need, and it won't be toxic.

And so, only ten or so generations ago, the best our forebears could manage for concentrated sweetness was a bit of honey if they were lucky, together with eating whatever ripe fruit they could get their hands on in the short period those fruit were in season.

The odd King or Queen or Emperor and their courts might have been able to get sweet things year round, but that was it. And okay, you got me, there *is* a fair bit of historical evidence that Henry VIII must have had a large barrel of honey-glazed chicken wings stashed somewhere in Hampton Court at all times. But that was just him.

Then, along came the industrialisation of food production and food manufacturers soon realised something very quickly – the more sugar they could get into any food or drink, the more it sold! Why? Because that's the way our bodies are programmed. We seek out sweetness in food the same way a baby calf seeks out milk from its mother's teats. It's in our DNA, in our systems, part of our design.

The point is that from the time business got involved in food production onwards, more and more sugar was added to our food and drink in an ever more sophisticated fashion – and sometimes not-so-sophisticated.

How did Pepsi so successfully take on Coke? They added more sugar. How did Coke strike back? It added more sugar still! Ah, but Pepsi got them in the end, as a can of their stuff is now 41 grams of sugar, while Coke is a mere 39.75 grams.

In Australia, how did Tim Tams blow Milk Arrowroot biscuits off the shelves, from 1964 onwards? They had over *four* times as much sugar in each biscuit! (Not to mention heaps more fat, and chocolate!)

But herein came the big problem, and I do mean *big*.

Because while suddenly getting so much sugar into our system might have felt great for us, our bodies simply are not designed to be overloaded with so much sweetness and they rebel against it.

The problem became all the greater from the 1820s on, when the newly forming food industry worked out how to mass produce that thing you and I know as table sugar.

What they did was take sugar cane, pulp it, and remove every last ounce of fibre from it, leaving only the sugary syrup which could then be laced into many other food products on a scale previously unimagined. With that, sugar consumption began to climb, spreading far beyond the Royal Court, as everyone started to eat like kings, and it went up even further in the late 1800s when products like Coke and chocolate took off. By 1900, average sugar intake in the Western world was about 15 grams a day.

It climbed further still after the Second World War when home refrigeration enabled these things called supermarkets to prepare meals that could be taken home for later consumption – most of them laced with sugar – which was also the time that sugar-filled breakfast cereals became the 'breakfast of champions', and everyone else besides.

And then, from about 1975 onwards, sugar consumption exploded in the Western world, particularly with the American discovery that instead of pulping sugar cane to get your sugar, the same could be done by pulping corn to make, after a long process, corn syrup – a substance even more laden with fructose than table sugar, easier to transport to food factories, and about half as expensive to produce! What is more, Lustig notes, if you give table sugar a value of 100 on your sweetness scale, then high fructose corn syrup comes in at 120! (Glucose comes in at a comparatively moderate 74.)

Bingo. Corn syrup made its way into even more products than standard sugar had already got to, and at much higher levels, meaning fructose consumption increased alarmingly . . . as did obesity levels.

(This, despite the fact that, in the US, still pursuing the theories of Ancel Keys, fat consumption had dropped significantly . . . Time had told the story. With the public health focus on fat, not sugar, Americans had still got ever bigger, diabetes among adults had shot up, even while the Journal of the American Medical Association in 2007 noted an extraordinary surge in Type 2 diabetes among youth in the United States, which, just a decade before, had been practically unknown.

In Australia, the explosion of diabetes is completely horrifying:[1]

A disease practically unknown in 1980 now affects around one million Australians.

It got to the point that, today, average sugar consumption is around 105 grams a day, while teenage boys in

75

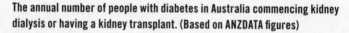

The annual number of people with diabetes in Australia commencing kidney dialysis or having a kidney transplant. (Based on ANZDATA figures)

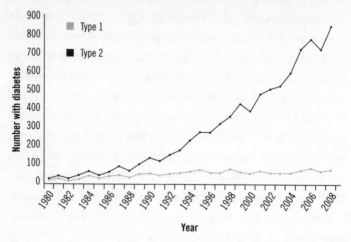

particular, who guzzle soft drinks and the like, can be putting 134 grams and more through their system per day.

You see, corn syrup is really so cheap that, as an example, and as documented by Robert Lustig in his 2009 lecture, the food companies doing business in Texas were able to come together so that they could market three products together in what they called a Big Gulp – 60 ounces of Coca-Cola (about 1.75 litres), a Snickers bar and a bag of Doritos all for 99 cents. As Lustig notes, 'If you did that every day for a year, that would be worth [51 kilograms] of fat per year.'

Such devastating consequences occur because, as Yudkin, Lustig and other researchers have established, while fructose tastes wonderful – and is in fact twice as sweet as glucose – it circumvents the usual process where our bodies break down other carbs into glucose, the blood sugar our bodies use as fuel.

Thinking again of our model of the tummy as the main tank, and the flab around it as the rubbery reserve tank, fructose does not act as a source of energy for the main tank. We eat fructose in sugar, with glucose. Glucose fills the main energy tank. Fructose is redundant and, just like alcohol, it's broken down by the liver, transformed into fat and goes into our bloodstream as circulating fat – becoming your bad cholesterol – before settling into our reserve tank as flab. In the face of what appears to be that rare moment of harvest time, with suddenly sweet, mature fruit on offer, we are programmed to act as if this is the one chance we'll get to get some fat on us before the winter, so we gorge, and all excess goes to fat. Our only hope of reducing that flab is that the body burns through everything in the main tank first, and then gets to it.

Fat chance!

The second thing the scientists on the Yudkin side of the argument established was that the fructose stuffed up the whole system of our bodies telling us when we've had enough, via the aforementioned fuel gauge in our brain. In fact, worse than that, not only does it not tell us we have had enough, it tells us we need *more*! And more and more and more . . .

Beyond suppressing the appetite-suppressant hormones of insulin and leptin – which tell us when we're full – fructose also uplifts the net level of another hormone called ghrelin, which comes from our stomach, and is the one which tells us we are hungry!

(With me, Boomka? In terms of the effect that it has on our bodies, on our stomach, our liver, our fat reserves, and our desire to keep eating more, fructose is what eminent scientists with the capacity to use any number of huge and incomprehensible words, in fact carefully define as a 'cluster-fuck'.)

If you can't burn it straight off, how much fat does it produce? A very rough approximation is, about a gram of fat for every four grams of sugar you see on the back of the label.

Think on that, next time you want to guzzle a Coke. At 39 grams of sugar, that one Coke is going to put about ten grams of fat into your reserve tank – even before it makes you hungrier so you consume more crap. And if you want to know what our livers can become like, think of *foie gras*. When I lived in provincial France in the mid-1980s, playing rugby, I saw up close how the farmers force-fed their geese, as this made their livers fatty, producing delicious foie gras and that, broadly, is what happens to our livers by putting too much sugar through them.

This is because the fructose does weird things to the two principal appetite-control hormones discussed before. While the pancreas releases insulin in response to the glucose in our blood, and insulin is an appetite suppressant, fructose causes *no* release of insulin and therefore doesn't suppress our appetite at all! If you ate pure fructose you would *never* feel full.

I know, I know, it is very easy to get lost in all this, and if you like, skip this bit and just take away the absolute key thing you need to know: sugar roots your system, and beyond piling on the calories, it makes you ever hungrier.

If you *do* want to get to the bottom of it, though – and it took me a while – the best explanation came to me in an email from Professor Alejandro Gugliucci, in response to my earnest enquiries. I am paraphrasing, but what he said was this: The glucose half of sugar produces insulin, which helps fill our tank with energy we can draw on, stored first in our muscles and in our liver. The excess glucose and all the excess fructose makes fat – in the blood, in our liver, on our stomach. Now, every time we take a huge load of sugar into our system, our blood sugar spikes high and we produce a surge of insulin to deal with it. Effectively, the insulin is SHOUTING to our brain: we have high glucose in our blood and need all hands on deck to remove it, and get it into storage. Over time, the brain becomes deafened by all the shouting and becomes progressively more 'insulin resistant'. And when it can't hear the insulin properly – compounded by the fact that the brain also becomes deaf to leptin – it inclines us to keep eating. The pancreas, meanwhile, in the hope of being heard, keeps turning up the volume of insulin. With the insulin resistance, your body now needs between two to five times more insulin than it did, to keep your blood sugar at normal levels, all while the insulin resistance, the brain deafness, is making us eat more and get fatter, and lifting our blood pressure.

'You keep putting on more weight,' Professor Gugliucci noted to me, 'until the pancreas gives out . . . and you're diabetic. The fat in your blood, meanwhile, starts you on the way to having a heart attack.'

Ugly as a hatful, isn't it?

To return to my own, rather more gauche metaphor, the fuel we put in our body can only cope efficiently with a certain amount of sugar in it – and for maximum efficiency, to have our motor purring and a real tiger in our tank, we should have no more than six to nine teaspoons a day. Any more than that is bad news. But if we put multiples of that amount in, the motor and the whole system is soon buggered. We just keep pouring that shit into our reserve tank, and when the needle on our fuel gauge doesn't tremble, we just keep pouring and pouring, getting bigger and bigger until something's got to give – either our pants, our pancreas, our heart or our brain, with a stroke.

Our motor seizes with the sugar, just as surely as German tanks and trucks seized back in the Second World War when the partisans of the mighty French Resistance used to sneak up on them in the darkness and pour sugar into their petrol tanks. Only a few hours into the next day, just when they were on the charge, the motors on the tanks and trucks would splutter and die, and they were rooted until the whole fuel, carburettor and piston system could be flushed out.

The key to the whole thing is that the fructose half of sugar gets a free pass to enter the system, without making us full, despite going straight to fat.

In terms of changing what I ate and drank, my own lightbulb moment came with understanding that when

I habitually knocked back a couple of cups of apple 'juice' that I always had before most commercial domestic flights, it had the caloric equivalent of five – count 'em, FIVE – apples. If, instead of the juice, I'd had those five apples I likely couldn't have eaten a bite of lunch. But when those calories came with a sugar hit, not only did it have none of the nutritional value of apples, but it all went straight to fat and the sugar hit made me twice as hungry as I would otherwise have been!

I have not had one of those small cups of concentrated sugar since.

I should make clear that none of Yudkin, Lustig, Gugli-ucci, Gillespie *et al* give fat a free pass. Not one of them says it's okay to pile into fatty foods at all. Their point is that if you have the fatty food with the sugar, you just keep piling into both, and do not have a natural mechanism to stop, to tell you when you are full – and so you inevitably over-eat. Because the body can no longer read the fuel gauge properly, we eat ever more food before we get that full feeling, and so just keep getting fatter.

Without the sugar, though, everything works the way it should and we stop over-indulging.

Yudkin himself conducted a study which demonstrated that when people were put on a diet with the only caveat being that they have no carbohydrates, while quaffing as much fat and protein as they liked, they actually cut their overall intake of calories by a third!

Without sugar boosting their hunger to a level far beyond what their bodies needed, they ended up self-regulating, and eating much less fat, too. Consequently, they all lost weight.

Now, while dry dissertations about the biochemical properties of sugar at a molecular level made my head hurt, the key prediction that Gillespie made, that if I knocked out the sugar, I'd stop the hunger, eat commensurately less, and lose weight . . . proved to be *100 per cent correct.*

MAGIC.

And I place my 45 kilograms lost, and kept off, up against all the nonsense diets and solutions above in Chapter Three – and even the sensible ones like the CSIRO diet.

Yes, beyond losing sugar from my diet, I added two other significant things – which I'll get to – but knocking sugar out was the key to unlocking this new world of health. I wish I'd come across it decades ago. Not only that, but so many of my aforementioned readers, who read my original article on weight loss, embraced the ideas, and knocked out the sugar for starters, have come back to me since, reporting that has been exactly their experience, too.

Once they stopped the sugar, the hunger stopped, they ate less and lost weight.

If you embrace this, you are *not* going on a diet. You and I both know that diets are tedious. You are *changing* your diet.

And this bloody thing works!

Got it?

One more time!

Blah, blah, blah.

Stop the sugar and you stop the hunger!

Blah, blah, blah.

SIX

Weaning yourself off sugar

'When I gave up sugar it was amazing. It was like pushing a toboggan along a track to eventually get down the slope. The first couple of weeks, the first couple of months, early May through June [was hard]. By the time I get to July and August we're going downhill and the weight's just coming off me . . .'
Alec Baldwin, actor

'If you removed all items containing sugar from a supermarket's shelves, just 20 per cent of items would remain.'
Damon Gameau, writer and director of *That Sugar Film*

'Fructose pulls a real two-card trick on our digestive system. Its calories sneak past undetected, giving us permission to

eat more. The undetected fructose gets converted directly to fatty acids and then those fatty acids degrade our ability to tell when we are full, giving us permission to eat even more.'
David Gillespie, author

'It is a biological error to confuse what a person puts in their mouth with what it becomes after it is swallowed. The human body, far from being a passive vessel for whatever we choose to fill it with, is a busy chemical plant, transforming and redistributing the energy it receives.'
Ian Leslie, British journalist

While it's one thing to decide to get off sugar, it is quite another to be able to work out in which food and drink the damaging substance can be found, and then actually change your diet to avoid it.

And yes, it is a little more difficult than no longer putting sugar in your coffee, sprinkling it on your Weet-Bix or buying packets of it from the supermarket. For, of course, the truly staggering thing is just how many other foodstuffs, beyond the obvious, boast that white stuff . . . even the food we don't think of as sweet!

So the first question to be asked is, how do you tell what food has sugar in it?

Well, the answer is that it is a little like that old gag:

Question: 'How do you know when a politician is lying?'
Answer: 'You can see his lips moving!'

In the case of food, it would go something like this.

Question: '*How do you know if packaged food has sugar
        in it?*'
Answer: '*Because it's packaged food!*'

And yes, there are exceptions, but that broad rule applies. If it's a product, as opposed to produce, it means it has been through the industrial food wringer, and just about *always* has sugar added to it on the way through!

Remember, big-business food and drink production don't get to be serious and profitable big businesses unless they sell their stuff in bulk, and they usually don't get to sell in bulk unless they put in it the siren call to food consumers the world over: **sugar**.

One of the documentaries put out by the Science Channel of National Geographic, *The Secrets of Sugar*, notes that the food industry has a short-hand term for just how much sugar, fat and salt they should put into their products, to maximise the craving of the consumers and the company's subsequent profits, which is called 'the bliss point'[1] with the salt covering for the sugar, which is high; the sugar covering for the salt, which is high. The salt and sugar make sure it doesn't taste too fatty, even though it is – and your body just knows it is getting *heaps* of all of them and wanting more, more, more!

To understand more on this, and to get a feel for just how much we consumers are coerced into buying and eating this 'food', google 'bliss point' and '*New York Times*', and read the feature story, *The Extraordinary Science of Addictive Junk Food*, by Michael Moss.

Read it and weep.

Mate, we've been played for mugs, and we've been eating like three mugs!

In terms of the sugar part of the bliss point, in few areas is it worse than breakfast cereals which, to my amazement, can be made up of just about a third sugar! Seriously, they don't call 'em 'cereal killers' for nothing.

And yes, mate, I know you think that the particular breakfast cereal *you* like is different, and healthy – just like they promise on the box and in the TV ads – and probably very low in sugar, but, one more time, you have to get a grip.

Even things like Uncle Tobys Oats Berry & Nut – which *looks* like a perfectly healthy product – is 23 per cent sugar.[2] So, switch to Kellogg's Sultana Bran, then, as bran is good for you, and sultanas are a healthy fruit? No. That is 22.7 per cent sugar.[3] This is representative of a huge problem – so many foods marketed as healthy are in fact loaded with sugar.

On this 'un, the advertising industry positively outdoes itself with its creative licence. My favourite of the genre was a couple of years ago, when Ironman champion Ky Hurst was flogging Nutri-Grain.

Here is Ky, on the beach, looking a million dollars, as he trains at dawn, on his way to becoming first an Ironman champion and then an Olympian. He gives to his sport, he tells us, '110 per cent'.

Don't lecture ME, Ky! Did I mention *I* was once leading Grant Kenny and Guy Leech after five rounds of a heptathlon on a *60 Minutes* special on Who Is Australia's Fittest Athlete?

But yes, I guess, you may as well tell everyone else . . .

So spruik for your life, Ky, while we look at the glorious slo-mo of your rippling lean body in action: 'I've trained hard, and achieved incredible success because, to be an Olympian, you only get out what you put in.'

Cut to vision of Ky eating Nutri-Grain. 'Kellogg's Nutri-Grain, where could it take you?' he finishes as the music rises to a crescendo.

The short answer is – as no less than 32 per cent of Nutri-Grain was pure sugar at the time the ad was made – it would most likely take you to the hospital, in a *crescendo* of sirens, pausing only at the clothing store to get bigger clothes because you're now so FAT.

I repeat: *32 per cent sugar!*[4,5]

F. F's. Sake!

The equivalent would be if you gave your child, say, two cups of oats for breakfast, and add roughly eight teaspoons of sugar on top.

Dare I say that you would be unlikely to produce an Olympic champion on that? Can I go further and say if at the table next to you at a cafe, you saw a mother or father give their kids a bowl of oats and then added eight teaspoons of sugar you'd consider it something very close to child abuse? At least, in 2015, in response to the uproar, Kellogg's reduced the sugar in Nutri-Grain to 27 per cent. That will make ALL the difference!

And the vast majority of such breakfast cereals are the same. I do mean most mueslis, too. Bear in mind, the original recipe for muesli, says Wikipedia, is: 'Two or three small apples or one large one, grated. Nuts, either walnuts, almonds, or hazelnuts, one tablespoon. Rolled oats, one tablespoon, previously soaked in 3 tablespoons water for 12 hours. Lemon juice from half a lemon.'[6] We've come a long way, baby.

Compare this with the 'Toasted Muesli Recipe' from Taste.com: '1/4 cup honey, 1/4 cut brown sugar, 1/4 cup olive oil, 3 cups rolled oats, 1/2 cup bran flakes, 1/2 cup flaked coconut, 1/4 cup sunflower seeds (Editor, this may be a typo, sounds healthy), 1/4 cup chopped pecan nuts, 1/2 cup dried apple, 1/2 cup dried cranberries.'

Most commercial mueslis are equally packed with sugar.

Straight out oats, however, are the honourable exception – around one per cent sugar only.

Oh, and that fruit juice you love to have with it, the really, really healthy one that comes from the big plastic bottle?

Disaster, mate. Absolute, card-carrying disaster. Think Chernobyl! Add the 2015 Ashes campaign . . . and throw in the time you told your missus, 'You know what . . . your bum *does* look a bit big in that!'

For what have they done to get that juice? They have taken the whole beautiful fruit, pulped the living daylights out of it, and then removed the fibre, the pulp, which is what contains so much of the actual goodness and nutritional value of the fruit to begin with. All that's left over is the sugary syrup – liquid sugar, if you will, primed to convert into flab quicker than anything else you can consume!

All up, at seven teaspoons of sugar in a 100 gram bowl of, say, Nutri-Grain – 'cos we both know you have well over double the mere handful that the 'usual' serving size of 40 grams is – and six teaspoons in a glass of fruit juice, and two teaspoons of sugar in your coffee, you have, simply at breakfast:

1. Eaten 12 times as much sugar as our forebears ate in a whole day and 25 per cent more than the World Health Organization's recommended maximum daily dose for an adult male.[7]
2. Converted 64 grams of sugar to 248 calories, which, if you don't burn off (and you won't), goes straight to your reserve tank – read, your belly. Even more problematic, it lifts your blood fat, giving you a heightened level of bad cholesterol and settles on your liver. Dr Lustig and Professor Gugliucci have done studies on obese American children, who get a quarter of their calories from sugar, and found that, in Professor Gugliucci's words, 'many have fatty livers comparable with the worst adult drunks'.
3. Sated your hunger only briefly, before all the sugar burns up in an hour or two, making you mid-morning ravenous for . . . *more* sugar.

And that's just for breakfast! Have a look at the muffin you have for morning tea. About eight teaspoons of sugar.

Washed down by a Coke, a further nine teaspoons.[8] And let's not forget the slice of birthday cake handed out at the office, because Cheryl from Accounts has turned 30 – eight teaspoons. The mid-afternoon creamy cappuccino pick-me-up, which you sweeten with another two teaspoons of sugar. The Kit Kat you buy at the service station on the way home, three teaspoons.

A dinner of pasta with a nice sugary spaghetti sauce straight from the bottle, five teaspoons. And apple pie and ice-cream for dessert, add another eight teaspoons. Mate, it's just been a normal day, and somehow, you've knocked back 58 teaspoons of sugar, which is to say nearly a quarter of a kilo of sugar! Listen, on that diet, which you and I know might even look like a light day for you when you're at your worst, you are putting through your system just shy of two kilograms of sugar every freaking week!

As you can now see, if you took the sugar content from the food the average Australian family with two kids has in just a week, it would add up to over four kilos.

The point is, that to go sugar-free it really does take some time to get your head around just how much of a pandemic sugar is, how prevalent it is in so many foods we were never aware of, and a few we suspected all along. But all of them are shocking.

Butterscotch – 81 per cent sugar.

Maple syrup – 68 per cent sugar.

Cranberry sauce – 38 per cent sugar.

Milo – 47 per cent sugar.

Tasmanian Crunchy Dried Apple Wedges – 76 per cent sugar!

Dried apricots – 34 per cent sugar.

Mint sauce – 36 per cent sugar.

Kellogg's Honey Smacks – 56 per cent sugar.

Vaalia Low Fat French Vanilla Yoghurt – 15 per cent sugar.

Fruit smoothies – 59 per cent sugar.

Powerbar energy bars – 36 per cent sugar.

Raisins – 72 per cent sugar.

Tomato sauce – 32 per cent.

Masterfoods BBQ sauce – 54 per cent.

Tim Tams – 44 per cent.

You get it?

The first thing is, don't believe the advertising images, particularly when it comes to trying to work out what is and isn't healthy. (And next time you're at a sausage sizzle, or outside Bunnings, think about the advisability of plastering your white bread and greasy sausage with a commercial paste that is OVER ONE-HALF sugar!)

Another recent ad that comes to mind is the one by Olympic swimmer Eamon Sullivan, where, standing shirtless in the kitchen, he showed off his perfect abs, as he baked with CSR sugar. The message of the ad is that if you bake with sugar, you, too, will end up with a body like Sullivan's, whereas – respectfully to him – a fairer representation would be to have *MasterChef*'s Matt Preston go shirtless, as he flogs the product.

The point is, that to avoid all this, it is not as simple as looking for products boasting 'No added sugar', or 'Contains only natural sugars'. That is marketing *schtick* that could mean anything! The question is not just how much sugar is added to it, champion, but how much sugar was in it to begin with?

Have a look at the label. One bottle of Coles 100% Apple Mango Juice No Added Sugar has five teaspoons per serving,[9] meaning that, despite its seeming 'healthy' appearance, it is in fact little more than sugar in a glass!

But . . . but . . . but the sugar in the apple juice is 'natural', you say? Look, on one level, so is the sugar in the can of Coke, derived as it is from either sugar cane or corn. That is no argument. The body does not care where the fructose molecule started life – from an apple picked yesterday, or from sugar cane harvested two years ago. For fructose is fructose is fructose. And it's killing us.

Incidentally, be equally wary of food advertising itself as Low Fat, Fat Free, 98 per cent Fat Free, etc. For starters, reflect on the fact that when a rich glob of 100 per cent fat is placed in a glass of water it, too, is now in a container that is '98 per cent fat free'!

More often than not, all those claims can be translated as Shitloads of Sugar, because that is precisely what the manufacturers have whacked into it to give it the secret lure that the fat used to.

Among the worst of these are the very popular smoothies, in the image of Gloria Jean's 98 per cent fat free Mango Fruzie, which in large size actually has – and this shocks even me – an extraordinary 123 grams of sugar in it, which is to say 31 teaspoons' worth![10] You'd need to drink 1.2 litres of Coke to get the same amount . . .

Shocking, yes?

Double ditto on so much of what is marketed as 'health food'.

Like, if tonight on the way home, instead of getting a Kit Kat, you get a standard muesli bar, do you think that might fix everything? Maybe eat two, to be doubly healthy?

Think again. Have a look on the back of it, mate, where the label is. Even an Uncle Tobys Muesli Bar (a fruit one, not a chocolate one) is just under 20 per cent sugar! As noted in *That Sugar Film* – which is well worth watching to widen and deepen your understanding of all this – 'People think if they give their children a muesli bar it is a healthy snack, but in reality they may as well be giving them a Mars bar.'

Blokes trying to steer away from sugar also often fall into the trap of steering away from obviously sugary snacks at the checkout, and going for the likes of chips instead. Don't. I quote the aforementioned authoritative article in the *New York Times* on the subject of the extraordinary science of junk food: 'The coating of salt, the fat content that rewards the brain with instant feelings of pleasure, the sugar that exists not as an additive but in the starch of the potato itself – all of this combines to make [chips] the perfect addictive food.' The article quotes Harvard Professor Eric Rimm: 'The starch is readily absorbed. More quickly even than a similar amount of sugar. The starch, in turn, causes the glucose levels in the blood to spike – which can result in a craving for more.'

And who can doubt it? Isn't that your experience with your first salt and vinegar chippie? Who can stop at a couple of chips? Mate, in this realm, we are simply outgunned by food scientists who are much smarter than we are. The only way to beat them is to just stay away from that shit in the first place – and the truth is, you quickly lose your taste for it.

Look, if you can grasp all this, and kick the need for sugar, you will look back on the sheer insanity of your diet – just as I did – and seriously wonder why you and I could ever have been so bone-stupid as to swallow all that marketing crap, let alone wallow in such sugar-soaked offal as part of our diet.

Looking back, the worst of it was when you and I used to go to Maccas and wash down the Big Mac, Filet-o-Fish and large fries with a large Coke – at least I did, and regularly at that.

Sometimes, if I spoke at a lunch in Canberra, on the drive back to Sydney I'd stop off at the Maccas just north of Goulburn and have exactly that meal, before making it home in time for dinner! And even speaking at a dinner there, I could stop off for a late-night bite and guzzle!

Didn't I used to see you there?

But with that meal, we were tipping down our gullet 600 millilitres of carbonated sugar-water containing no less than 55.1 grams of sugar – 14 teaspoons! – of which 27.5 grams are fructose, converting to 12 grams of body fat, as we sit at the wheel.

And even then, the damage was only just starting, as the Coke made us hungrier still, and even more inclined to buy more junk food from the same outlet! (Funny that.)

Yes, we could burn it off, but just to get rid of the calories gained from that large Coke, we're talking the need to walk briskly for 45 minutes!

And who actually *does* that? Does extra exercise to burn off excess calories?

Most people don't. They just get ever fatter as the years go by.

Sad, isn't it, how some blokes let themselves go?

Thank gawd you and I have stopped.

Because now we know: drinking that shit is MADNESS. And if you are giving it to your kids – just like I sometimes did at Maccas when my wife wasn't with us, before I knew better – I reckon, that, too, is perilously close to child abuse.

You heard me.

And I did it. (Ssshh, do *not* tell your mother, or we won't come again.)

At the least it is wilful ignorance. Whatever else, feeding that shit to your kids is putting convenience ahead of health.

So what should you be eating instead?

Let's start with a healthy breakfast.

If you want a bowl of something, unflavoured porridge with no sugar is a good place to start. Or sugar-free, fruit-free, untoasted muesli can be excellent. A couple of Australian mobs I've come across make it in bulk – and they seem to be down-home sort of people. Try googling Flips Muesli or The Muesli Club. My wife, meantime, swears by something called 'The Good Mix, Blend 11', which comes,

I gather, from an equally valiant small Australian business, making 100 **per** cent natural food.

These days, for what it's worth, after much experimentation as to what is the best breakfast for me, I have settled on having a couple of poached eggs, half a sliced avocado and some mushrooms.

For lunch I try to have some version of a chicken salad, and dinner more often than not is fish or grilled chicken, or often a large salad with no meat at all in it, but perhaps a bit of tuna. (More on salads and recipes in a later chapter.)

The amazing thing? After going sugar-free, I just don't *want* to eat the huge slabs of bacon and red meat I used to get by on for breakfast, lunch and dinner. That is because my whole palate has changed, across the board.

And yes, early on, of course I had sugar cravings that I had to fight.

A Tim Tam? No, thank you, I really . . . couldn't.

Dessert, dear? I actually don't think I will . . . tonight.

But I got there.

And you'll know you've got there, too, when instead of having the daily struggle of trying to stop yourself eating and drinking crap, there is no struggle at all because you just don't want that stuff anymore, but rather, actively want good food and drink.

Do you get it? Once you lose your taste for sugary crap, everything else starts to come good. You change your whole mind-set from *these are the things I can't eat on this diet, these are the things I must pull back on . . . even though I really want them . . .* which is a TEDIOUS way to live.

And instead you move into ... *these are the healthy foods I really* DO *want to eat*, which is a joy.

Instead of trying to follow all these rules and regulations which come with most diets – which, as you know, is perilously close to that worst of all possible things, Un-Australian! – you move into a new space.

Instead of restrictions and deprivations, you guzzle with gusto and tuck in with fervour – but on good things.

So, where do you find those good things? One quick ready-reckoner is that they are mostly found on the outside perimeter of the supermarket, where the fresh meat, fresh milk, fresh vegetables and fresh fruit are generally in position. The rest of the supermarket is packaged, processed and broadly unnatural – as in, full of sugar. (If you need any encouragement to stay away from the stuff in packets, understand that – far from being renewed daily on the shelves and in the bins like the fresh food – much of it is so packed with preservatives, it can last for as long as two years. Some of those biscuits, as Kenny the plumber might say, 'will outlast religion'.)

Fast food, too. A woman in Alaska, owner of a chiropractic clinic, made headlines in early 2016 by posting a photo online of a McDonald's Happy Meal she bought six years earlier – a burger, fries and chicken nuggets, marketed to kids – which showed no signs of aging.

'It's been six years since I bought this "Happy Meal" at McDonald's,' she wrote. 'It's been sitting at our office this whole time and has not rotted, molded, or decomposed at all!!! It smells only of cardboard. We did this experiment to show our patients how unhealthy this "food" is. Especially for our growing children!! There are so many chemicals in this food! Choose real food! Apples, bananas, carrots, celery . . . those are real fast food.'[11]

But, back to the supermarket.

If you insist on staying with some packaged food, at least learn to read the labels and work out what is and isn't loaded with sugar. There can be huge differences, just within the same basic food group.

As an example, while Tamar Valley yoghurt has 5.6 grams of sugar per 100 gram serve, Dairy Farmers Yoghurt has 15 grams. A broad rule is that while natural yoghurt has 5 grams of sugar (from the lactose in the milk), flavoured ones generally add at least 6 grams of extra sugar per 100 grams.

Frûche dessert, meanwhile, has 23 grams of sugar per serve!

Mate, whatever solution you come up with, the absolute key is to establish a routine, a system of living, a framework whereby you don't think about what you're having for breakfast, lunch and dinner, you *know* what you're having: one of several healthy options all predicated on the notion that 'healthy' relies on them having bugger-all sugar.

Equally, you don't go into morning tea and afternoon tea trying to muster the willpower to hold off on having a biscuit or two.

You don't *eat* biscuits anymore, remember? You're not a 'tea'-totaller, you're a biscuit-totaller, and part of the point of the exercise is to lose the taste for something that is killing you, just like you lost the taste for tobacco. What really helped me was going wall-to-wall for a while, on that sugar-free muesli mentioned above, just so I could give my system a chance to kick in, freshen up and apply its own diktats as to what I did and didn't want.

You need to have something on hand for when you get the munchies. Out goes the biscuit tin and the tray of muffins. Enough with the glazed donuts – dietary suicide. Gillespie suggests a jar of unsalted macadamias, cashews or almonds, and they have worked well for me. See, if you haven't got sugar in you to stuff up your fuel gauge it doesn't matter that much, because every calorie is being counted and when you get to dinner time, you won't be that hungry and will eat less accordingly. Yet another quick snack I love is a couple of teaspoons gouged out of an avocado – just enough to give Lisa the raging shits – before putting it back in the fridge. One day, I reckon they'll find avocado is the wonder food of our time. Just two mouthfuls and you're fine!

I also find that helping myself to a couple of spoonfuls of sugar-free muesli whenever I feel peckish helps heaps. Instead of those mid-morning or mid-afternoon pangs leading to a muffin or the like, loaded with sugar, washed down by a soft drink, equally loaded with sugar – all of which would contrive to make you ravenous by lunch or dinner – you just need something sugar-free to quell the pangs to see you through.

All up, the easiest way to get sugar out of your diet is to stay with just buying and preparing fresh food, but of course, sometimes that is not possible. Now, mostly, if you want to tell if a supermarket product has a lot of sugar in it, it is like working out if a Yank is a bit full of himself; if your wife is better than you deserve; and if the last time you were dropped from the top team it was a bit bloody unfair. Mostly, it just goes with the territory!

I repeat. I REPEAT:

If it is a 'product', as opposed to 'produce', as opposed to something that has come to you naturally, it pretty much *always* has sugar in it.

But, yes, there are some exceptions, and I cite specifically things like canned beans, frozen vegetables and pasta. The easiest and most foolproof way of finding out if what you're buying has sugar in it is to look on the back of the product. They are required by law to tell you exactly how much sugar is in it. Against that I reckon most manufacturers keep it in such impossibly small type and complex form that it must be designed to be indecipherable, and reading nutritional information on the back of packets still makes my head hurt. All those ingredients, all those percentages and stats. Plus, some of them trick you by, in my view, understating what a normal serving can be. Take Nutri-Grain for example. According to them, a normal serving is just 40 grams. Really? That is about a cup. Whoever has as little as that for brekka? Most adults, I believe, would have at least twice that for breakfast, meaning when they try to calculate how much sugar is in it, they must double what Nutri-Grain puts down on their label, as to grams of sugar per serving.

Truly, there is only one figure that need concern us. That is the number of grams under 'sugars' per 100 grams.

That, of course, will give you the percentage of sugar in it, and when you work out how many grams you're going to eat, you just need to divide the net grams of sugar by four to give yourself an approximation for how many grams of fat you're going to put in your reserve tank.

Now, do you *really* want those 100 grams of dried apples[12] you think are healthy, when in fact they have 57 grams of sugar, producing 14 grams of fat?

My own broad solution to navigate through all the mumbo-jumbo, away from the supermarket, is dead simple: 'Don't eat sweet.'

While your fuel gauge doesn't register the fructose, your tastebuds certainly can, so you *know* when it is in there!

And just as you might once have adored the smell of tobacco smoke, but now can't stand it, you can get to the same stage with sugar.

You know your life is better without smoking. I promise you it is better without sugar!

Now, to a few Frequently Asked Questions, as they say in the classics . . .

FAQ: Can I use honey as a sweetener for my food instead?

There's that word again: NO. And I know you think it is 'natural sugar', and therefore okay. But where do you think normal sugar comes from? Some lab, somewhere? What is sugar cane, if not natural? What is corn, if not natural? The only virtue of honey is that it is 40 per cent fructose, rather than 50 per cent for normal sugar,[13] but the difference is a bee's dick and the bottom line remains: sugar is sugar no matter where it comes from, and you gotta stop putting that shit in your system.

FAQ. How does not having sugar make you feel?

Not hungry! Seriously, once you try it, it is the revelation to beat them all. I know I keep banging on about it – and there is more to come – but it still stuns me that I got to the age of 50 without realising that this is the solution to the whole problem. Why on *earth* is this not broadcast far and wide?! You have a good and healthy breakfast without sugar, and you get to morning tea with no attack of the nibblies. You have a light and healthy lunch and have no interest in afternoon tea. You get to dinner, there is food on the table, but after you have had an 'elegant sufficiency', you push the plate away, wipe your mouth with your napkin, lean back, and look with pity on others ripping into the apple pie and ice-cream. You feel so superior, you can hardly STAND IT! You think you might even vote Liberal next election! And you get on the scales the next morning, and can barely believe it, but you have gone down. *Again.*

FAQ. Is it as hard as all get-out?

Not particularly for me, as it turned out. But some people reckon it can be as hard as giving up tobacco. They even note such unpleasant things as nausea and an upset tummy, not to mention being as grouchy as a bear with *two* sore heads, as they try to deal with the sheer craving. (But usually, Dr FitzSimons says, the worse the symptoms, the more

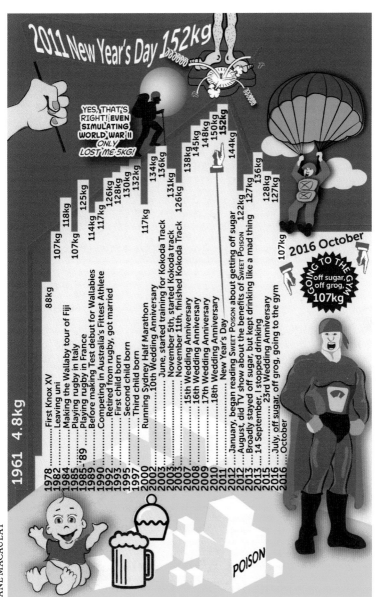

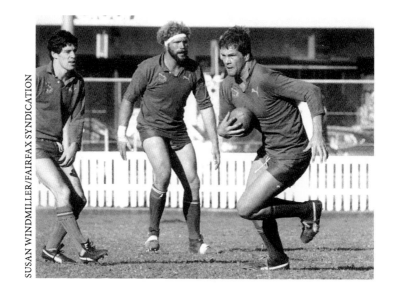

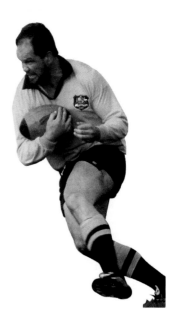

Playing days.

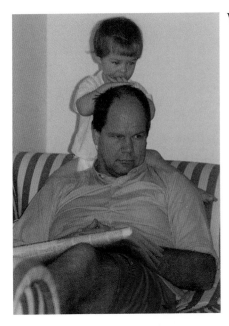

With Jake in 1996.

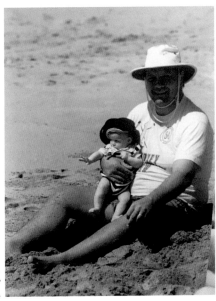

Christmas 1997,
Newport Beach.

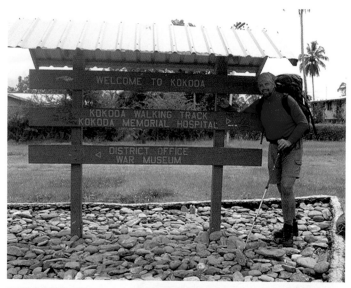

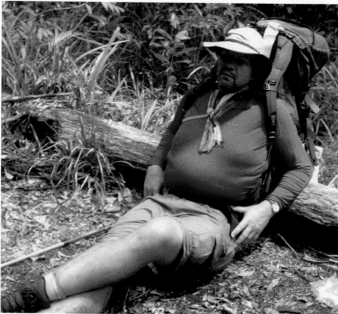

Kokoda Track, 2003.

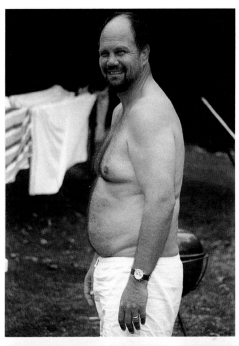

Christmas 2005.

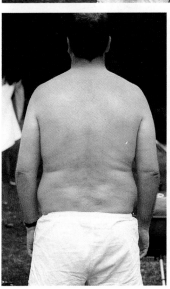

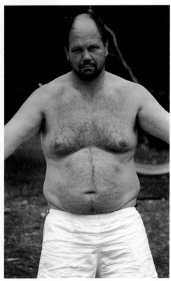

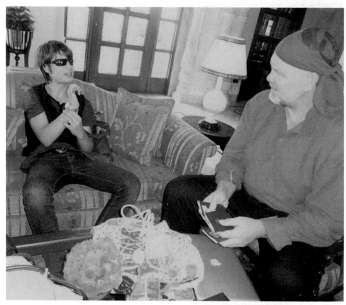

In 2007 with Louis.

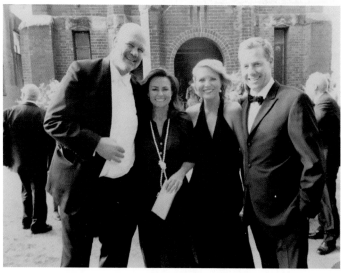

At a wedding with Lisa, Georgie Gardner and Ben Fordham, 2010.

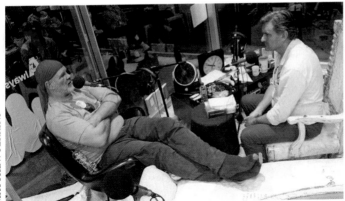

Breaking the Guinness world record for the longest one-on-one radio interview – 24 hours with Richard Glover, 2013.

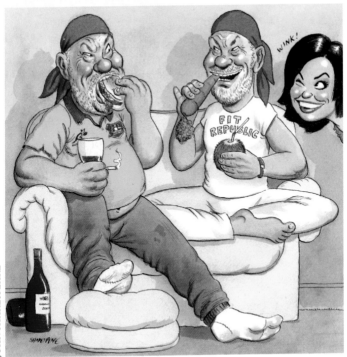

Cartoonist John Shakespeare's take on my change of diet.

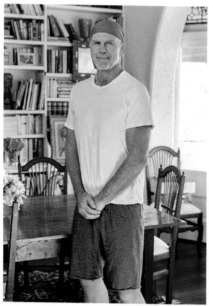

Me today.

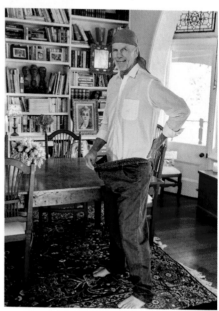

reason you need to give up the stuff. It's often symptomatic of your level of addiction.)

FAQ. How long does the craving last?

When I was a footballer, one of the running gags was that if you got a badly twisted ankle and received daily treatment on it, you could be back playing within a month, while with no treatment at all, it would take about four weeks . . .

Most people report the same amount of time for sugar cravings. After a month or so, you don't even think about it.

The key, for me, is that over time, my own 'bliss point' – of the ideal amount of sugar, salt and fat in food or drink to make it irresistible to eat – got progressively lower. That is, even when I would occasionally weaken and try a bit of a biscuit, I would spit it out as too sweet. And I might say, too fatty, as my tastes changed there, too. I no longer *want* it, any more than I wanted a drag on a Marlboro. My tastes have changed, become healthier, which takes all the pain out of trying to eat more healthily. At lunch, I don't have to think about it – I don't want dessert. At the service station, I am not being disciplined in not getting a Coke, ice-cream or Kit Kat or all of the above. I just, seriously, don't want them. Again, think how it was with sugar in your tea and coffee. Just persist through the craving part until you get to the clear air, where you simply don't want it anymore, and it's easy sailing from there on in!

FAQ. Is it difficult, socially, as in when you are invited to dinner and decline the hosts' dessert?

Occasionally, a bit. But something else to factor in is that people can get extraordinarily defensive when they realise you have different eating habits. It's a peculiar phenomenon, but people do feel threatened by alternative lifestyle choices. But, remember that ol' saying: 'To hell with the lot of 'em! Do it anyway!' This is your life. And you want to make it a long one. (Cue, my friend the comedian, Brian Doyle. 'When I die, I want to go peacefully, in my sleep, like my grandfather did. Not screaming and carrying on like all the people in the bus he was driving at the time.')

FAQ. Are there any pitfalls?

Yes. When, after three or four decades of getting bigger, you finally find the thing that turns it around and gives you back – and I used the word advisedly – your *youth*, you can get over-excited about it. You've discovered this thing, see, where simply by changing what you eat, and without ever going hungry, the weight just falls off you, mate, and you really should try it, mate, because I am telling you it is the best thing ever, and if you stop the sugar you drop the pud and the danger is . . . you NEVER SHUT UP ABOUT IT. (But if that is your case, let me at least sympathise. Once you twig on to this – that the whole obesity thing can be fixed so easily, just by changing your diet away from sugar – it is almost more than you can bear *not* to tell the miserable looking fat bloke next to you on the plane how he can sort the whole thing out, as an act of mercy. I try to stop myself being a proselytising prick about it, but as this book perhaps attests, in part, I do not always succeed.)

FAQ. But the reaction of friends is still a factor, yes?
Yes. It is as well to be aware of it: social pressure is a huge influence on our diets. But have a look around. Are those chipping you overweight? Sounds like breaking from the pack is exactly what you need! It's much too easy to cave in to the habits of your family/friends/colleagues and you dinkum do need to carve out your own space as to what you will eat and drink, entirely independent of what they are throwing down.

FAQ. After exercise and so forth, what do you drink instead of soft drinks?
Try . . . wait for it . . . WATER. Simple, beautiful, water. It is precisely what our body is *meant* to run on, and no amount of bells and whistles, additives, sugars, flavours etc, can make it any better for us than it already is. In fact, in *all* cases all the things added make it worse from a health perspective. And I include the sickly sweet Gatorade in that, in which one handy 'Thirst Quencher' bottle has nine teaspoons of sugar – marketed as being good for the health of athletes!

Take a Captain Cook.

Ditto, Powerade. Just one 600 ml bottle has about eight and a half teaspoons of sugar, meaning that, from the point of view of your body, it is the same as if you just sat down and ate 14 of those red frog lollies!

Look, I guess I should add a rider here that even Lustig does reluctantly note that for *elite* athletes, who've just run the likes of a marathon, these kind of drinks actually can replenish your glycogen stores more quickly, but it's the way he says 'elite' that makes me think he is not referring to you and me, Fatty.

You and I need water, and lots of it. Physiologically, the rule of thumb is that we need to sluice through our system, every day, one litre of water for every 33 kilograms of our mass. Drink up, son!

SEVEN

The politics of food

'As a culture, we've become upset by the tobacco companies
advertising to children, but we sit idly by while the food
companies do the very same thing. And we could make a
claim that the toll taken on the public health by a poor diet
rivals that taken by tobacco.'
Professor Kelly Brownell, Yale University

So, you've got the drift now, of both the perils of sugar and
how to avoid it? Great. Against all this, I need to offer a
word of warning. After I started spruiking the virtues of all
this in various forums in 2014 – most particularly on
Channel Seven's *Sunday Night* program, and in many
columns for Fairfax – I was amazed when I started taking
a little heat for taking off a lot of fat. I mean, shoot me, but
I thought this might be one of those unassailable good

news stories? I accept that it doesn't come close to the excitement of the Duchess of Cambridge opening a garden fete in a pretty dress, but in terms of putting your head above the parapet and inviting people to take a shot – which I do on many other subjects, like the republic, gun control, same-sex marriage, climate change, maintaining $10 million was too much to pay for Buddy Franklin etc., – it simply *never* occurred to me that my views on sugar could attract flak.

I mean, what are the bad things you could say about, 'Fat bloke, who used to be fit bloke, becomes fit and healthy again, and humbly offers clues to other fat blokes how they can become fit again too'?

Where, pray tell, is the downside?

Alas, no. I was to be exposed, even named and shamed, in *The Australian Women's Weekly*, in an article titled 'THE FIVE WORST CELEBRITY BACKED DIETS'. And by gawd, they didn't miss me *or* my mates, either:

'Eva Longoria, Megan Gale, Tom Hanks . . . Peter FitzSimons and Alec Baldwin are among high-profile followers of sugar-free diets.'

My goodness! How did they find out about us?

How did they *know*, that just three months earlier, while eating celery sticks down at the Carrot Club, there we were . . . Eva, Megan, Tommy, Smart Alec and me, standing around, lamenting lamingtons, decrying donuts and wondering just when our embarrassing pasttime of not loading up on sugar would be found out. Little did we know . . . the *Weekly* had already put their best and brightest on our tail, and were right onto us, as this particular story showed.

'People are looking for a prescription,' a Dietitians Association of Australia's spokesperson was quoted by the *Weekly*. 'But you can eat a healthy balanced diet including all food groups and lose weight. It's about cutting your portion sizes and getting outside and exercising.'

It actually also might help if, instead of the two kilograms a year of sugar that humans are equipped to eat without damage, we didn't have the 20 to 30 times that amount that so many of us do now. And if I know one thing from all this, it is that sugar is *not* just another 'food group'.

The DAA (that's the Dietitians Association of Australia, Boomka – acronymns are used throughout this book as they are very low in calories), mind, is the same organisation that, as documented by Gillespie, once put out a press release, titled 'Sweet truths: Eating sugar may not make you fat.'[1] I am serious! The Dietitians Association of Australia actually put out that press release because it was so important that Australians know that sugar is *not* the great white enemy!

Representing the DAA on the subject was their spokesperson, Dr Alan Barclay, who was the co-author of the study the press release was based on, a study that he had co-authored with Professor Jennie Brand-Miller, first published in the E-journal *Nutrients* that Dr Brand-Miller – from my own Sydney University, where I am a Fellow of the Senate – was guest editor of at the time.[2]

As the Kiwis say, the plot *thuckens* . . .

As Alan Barclay told the DAA conference, 'consumption of fructose has decreased by nearly 20 per cent in Australia since the early 1970s, while overweight and obesity has doubled'.

Odd.

'Much to everyone's surprise, it looks as if, unlike in the US, sugar is not the culprit here . . .'[3]

Ah-HA!

Now we are getting somewhere!

Enter the notorious 'Australian Paradox', which started out as a can of worms, but frankly more resembles – and I say this respectfully to all concerned – a nest of vipers, at least in terms of the hissing venom that has been hurled because of it.

The study purports to show that while 'research from the USA has demonstrated a positive relationship between sugars consumption and prevalence of obesity',[4] no such relationship exists here.

That is, while 'prevalence of obesity has increased three-fold in Australians since 1980 . . .' in this country, 'per capita consumption of refined sucrose decreased by 23% . . .'.

Yes, as Professor Brand-Miller would tell *The Australian*, even though 'Australians have been eating less and less sugar . . . rates of obesity have been increasing . . .'[5].

True! (Yes, here is the most paradoxical part of the 'Australian Paradox'.) Even as sugar consumption had declined, obesity levels had tripled!

In sum . . .

'The findings confirm an "Australian Paradox" – a substantial decline in refined sugars intake over the same timeframe that obesity has increased. The implication is that efforts to reduce sugar intake may reduce consumption but may not reduce the prevalence of obesity . . .'[6]

Who cares anyway, you say?

Well, Big Sugar in Australia does.

This report was manna from heaven to them, because from the moment that you can demonstrate in this country that the crippling rise in obesity – which saps the population of energy and the taxpayers' purse of funds for hospitals – is directly linked to an equivalent rise in sugar consumption, it is bleeding obvious that the duty of the Federal Government is to bloody well do something, starting with a sugar tax, to start to lower that consumption, and also to change their official dietary guidelines to encourage the population to consume less sugar.

But the Australian Paradox says that is not the case, that no such link can be established!

How could that be? While we all have our thinking caps on I think it fair to observe that the DAA's 'corporate partners' include Nestlé chocolate, Arnott's biscuits and Unilever, the maker of Street's ice-cream?[7] Over the years, such partners, and other food companies, have lent a helpful hand with the DAA's activities, with the likes of Kellogg's – purveyors of staggeringly sugary breakfast cereals – sponsoring the DAA's promotion of[8] Breakfast Week.[9]

Meanwhile the DAA's 2014 conference was *partly sponsored* by 'The Healthier Australia Commitment', which sounds great, until you realise they are an alliance of Nestlé, Coca-Cola South Pacific, Campbell Arnotts, Sugar Australia,

General Mills, Lion, Unilever and PepsiCo. What is wrong with this picture?

At another recent DAA conference, attendees were offered a free McDonald's Deli Choices Wrap, so long as they visited the Heart Foundation booth to get their food voucher and, sure enough, the Macca's Wrap had the tick of approval from the Australian Heart Foundation too.[10] (More on that, shortly.) Seriously, Dr Ronald McDonald is making a house call to the Dietitians conference? Does anybody at the DAA ever use the phrase, 'This is not going to look good' at conference planning meetings?

One of the features of the DAA website is an 'Accredited Practising Dietitian in the Spotlight'. Recently,[11] one dietitian they were bathing in warm attention proved to be the Director of Communications and Public Affairs at Kellogg's. Another was PepsiCo Australia's – and I am not making this up – 'Nutrition Manager'. (The mind boggles. And if you think your boss doesn't *care* what you think, try being the Nutrition Manager at PepsiCo!) Meanwhile, one of those on the board of the DAA is also the Director of the Australian Breakfast Cereal Forum of the Australian Food and Grocers Council.[12]

Now, and I mean this seriously, I don't call into question the integrity and professionalism of the individual dietitians who make up the membership of the DAA. I am actually close to several and know their dedication to the cause and the great work they do. But I can't help but wonder if the likes of Nestlé and Kellogg's and PepsiCo might be, just a bit, maybe, using the organisation of those dietitians, the

DAA, to make their products look a tad more healthy than they actually are? Friends, to my eyes, this is like developers getting themselves elected to local councils. Lots of those developers now running the show are lovely people, of impeccable integrity. But give them serious input into council deliberations on what the urban environment should look like, when the decisions they make for council affect their own profits? You can call me a visionary of stupendous wisdom if you like, but wouldn't it be better if they were one step removed.

And if you heard your local council was in a 'corporate partnership' with Big Bob's Development Inc, their motto being 'Every tree looks more beautiful with a block of flats on top of it', wouldn't you suggest to the council that it might look better, and be better, if they, like, DIDN'T DO THIS?

And I do say that any organisation devoted to promoting health that puts out pro-sugar press releases like 'Sweet truths: Eating sugar may not make you fat', which takes money from companies with that much sugar in their products, that has that level of integration between the companies and their organisation, has a case to answer.

If you care to google 'Rory Robertson and Australian Paradox' you will get a taste of just how strongly the Sydney economist – whose particular skill is picking apart statistics to discover truths – worked to help the DAA sleuths solve this puzzling 'Australian Paradox'. (Robertson, like me, had read Gillespie, dropped sugar out of his diet, and quickly and fairly effortlessly went from being a fat man to close to the weight he was when he was 20 and fit. Unlike me, he had an intellectual focus that would kill a brown dog, and was determined to find a solution to the paradox, which *has not shown up anywhere else in the world)*. Just to spell it out again for the slow Boomkas, here is the paradox, according to DAA members Dr Alan Barclay and Professor Jennie Brand-Miller. Everywhere else in the world people are eating more sugar and getting fatter. But in Australia, we're eating less sugar and getting fatter. A paradox!

Can you guess the solution?

Robertson is a fiend on the subject: the analysis of their data is wrong. Not just wrong in the sense of relying on out-of-date sugar consumption figures that – Robertson quickly discovered – the Australian Bureau of Statistics had *themselves* acknowledged as so unreliable they had stopped using them and in fact stopped gathering from 1999 on;[13] but some of the figures they used were wrong in the sense of being self-contradicting.

For instance, the paper stated that Australians were drinking ten per cent less sugary soft drink per capita now than in previous years, while also including a chart showing that consumption had risen by 30 per cent.[14] And Professor Brand-Miller had to admit that part of the report was wrong when interviewed on ABC radio, explaining, under some pressure, that a 'key word' had been left out of the report.[15]

But back to those paradoxical sugar consumption figures; Robertson actually went to the trouble of ringing some of the sources cited in 'The Australian Paradox' like ... the United Nations Food and Agriculture

Organization (FAO). Now, they sound like a wonderfully reliable collection of chaps and chapesses. And they are. Usually. But this time . . . well, it got interesting. You see, as he delights in recounting, they told him that they were relying on the Australian Bureau of Statistics figures! Rory told them those figures stopped being counted after 1999 because they were unreliable. The FAO confirmed with Rory that its 1999–2003 sugar figures for Australia – which feature in the 2011 Australian Paradox paper as a conspicuously dead-end, flat-line segment – are based on an algorithm, based on the last ABS figure published from 1999, not actual, real-world measurements . . .[16] You got it, Boomka. Rory insists they had reported figures that did not exist, based on an algorithm, based on figures so inaccurate that they were discontinued, that were then cited in an academic report . . .

For my money, we have found the solution to the 'Paradox'. And this silly sugar falsehood would have been on a self-perpetuating loop if the likes of Robertson had not called it out.

By analysing the figures from the Australian Bureau of Agricultural and Resource Economics – which is, in any case, precisely the kind of figures he has crunched through in his adult life to become a leading economist – Robertson contends that, in fact, in Professor Brand-Miller and Dr Barclay's own published chart, 'sugar availability' – based on figures from the Australian Bureau of Agricultural and Resource Economics – increased by about 20 per cent between 1980 and 2010.[17]

To be fair, as detailed by the ABC *Lateline* program in 2016, an external 'inquiry cleared Professor Brand-Miller and Dr Barclay of misconduct, but the report did observe that Dr Barclay's acceptance of a fee from Coca-Cola might not have demonstrated good judgement'.[18]

You can also read Brand-Miller and Barclay's robust defence of their position by googling, 'Trends in added sugar supply and consumption in Australia: there is an Australian Paradox . . .' Both have made it clear they will be saying more about it.

And I might note in passing, I do not accuse any of the aforementioned of misconduct either, and in any case am not remotely academically qualified to do so. But what I do believe, upon investigation, is that those scientists and academics who do hold such views can count on enormous support from the sugar companies, while a sure source of generous funding for those who want to ring alarm bells on sugar is not obvious.

Either way, if you google '*Lateline* and the Sugar Paradox', it completely demolishes the whole nonsense of the Paradox.

The dispute goes on, though it is worth noting that the dietitian with the most impeccable credentials in the country, Dr Rosemary Stanton of the University of NSW – who has graciously helped me a great deal with this book – has come down on the side of Robertson, in saying there is 'no evidence that sugar consumption in Australia has fallen and I have many objections to that particular paper and to the idea that sugar is not a problem'. For her part, Professor Brand-Miller has not backed off a jot, telling *Lateline* the findings in the Australian Paradox paper were more valid than ever.[19]

Personally, I remain more sceptical than ever. I just hope that health conscious companies PepsiCo and Kellogg's and Nestlé can form new corporate partnerships with people like Rory and others who want to ring alarm bells on sugar.

Still, the DAA is not alone when it comes to an influential health organisation steering us into very strange territory on the subject of sugar and our health.

The Australian Diabetes Council appear very careful not to point the finger of doom at sugar as one of the prime causes of diabetes.

Curious, Watson. I think this may be a three-pipe problem . . .

Meanwhile, the Head of Research for the Australian Diabetes Council from 1998 to 2014 – well, *hulloa!* – Dr Alan Barclay, steadfastly maintains, as he told the *Today* program, that the way to prevent diabetes is, in fact, to cut intake of fat and salt, while eating more fish. In that interview, mention of sugar – regarded by an ever-growing nucleus of scientists globally as a key cause of Type 2 diabetes – did not make the cut.

In June, 2016, Dr Barclay wrote an article for SBS, where he sought to correct two 'Myths'.

Myth 1: Sugar causes diabetes.

Myth 2: People with diabetes should not have sugar.[20]

The official position of the former Australian Diabetes Council – which recently changed its name to the Diabetes

Council of NSW – is the same, maintaining that 'We want to end the myth that sugar causes diabetes'.[21]

Now I am no fan of myths. (Except the one about when St George slayed the Loch Ness Monster with a golden thread before he turned into a pumpkin at midnight – that was a cracker.) But I, and plenty of people who actually know what they are talking about, was extremely surprised to find out that the link between sugar and diabetes was a myth. But let's go with it for the moment. What should diabetics eat then?

Well, the Diabetes Council's official recommendation is 'that people with diabetes choose at least one serve of a low G.I. food at each meal and snack'.[22]

Okay, good to know. To find out about dietary GI let's go over to the Glycemic Index Foundation, keepers of the medical construct that, very broadly, it is possible to form a 'relative ranking of carbohydrate in foods according to how they affect blood glucose levels'.

If only we had someone we knew to explain further . . .

Their spokesperson – goodness! – Dr Alan Barclay, maintains that losing weight and countering diabetes has nothing to do with the sugar that ill-educated nuts like I and the Mayo Clinic (more on them shortly) are obsessed with, either, and much to do with buying foods with ticks for Low GI.

Those foods include Nestlé Muesli Bars, with 25 per cent sugar, and Nestlé's Milo, with 47 per cent sugar.

Look, they could only be more dismissive of the effects of specifically fructose on diabetes sufferers if they endorsed a product that was 100 per cent fructose, correct? Well, they do. Danisco puts out a product called Fruisana Fruit Sugar 'the low GI alternative to cane sugar',[23] which, of course, comes with the Low GI tick of approval.

I know, I was stunned, too. And confused. How could something that is pure fructose – *the* killer nutrient identified by Lustig and scientists around the world as doing terrible damage to our health – get a big thumbs-up from the Low GI crowd, that the Diabetes Council had steered us to? And then I remembered, fructose is metabolised by your liver to fat, not glucose, so, whatever else, it doesn't mean there is an immediate spike in your blood sugar, so, according to Low GI people, all good.

In fact, Dr Alan Barclay and, yes, Professor Jennie Brand-Miller, are among co-authors of a book titled *Low GI Diet Diabetes Handbook*, which makes the extraordinary claim, 'There is absolute consensus that sugar in food does not cause diabetes.'[24]

This news did not reach Dr Stanton, who says, in a consensus-ruining response, 'The people who eat the most sugar have by far the highest risk of Type 2 diabetes. So I think that evidence is now compelling.'[25] And it is. In fact, in recent times, medical research has only cranked the siren up louder in warning of the dangers of sugar, especially sugared drinks, for Type 2, and many other health conditions for that matter, most particularly affecting the heart, liver and kidneys.

In 2015, the *British Medical Journal* – drawing on 17 previously published studies on links between sugary drinks and diabetes risk – found that drinking one sugar-sweetened beverage each day led to an 18 per cent increased risk of diabetes over a decade.[26]

In 2015, one of the most highly regarded medical establishments in the world, the Mayo Clinic, conducted a comprehensive review of all available animal and human trials on fructose and concluded: 'Added fructose in particular (e.g. as a constituent of added sucrose or as the main component of high-fructose sweeteners) may pose the greatest problem for incident diabetes, diabetes-related metabolic abnormalities, and [Cardio-Vascular] risk.'[27]

How is that 'absolute consensus' travelling now?

And yes, there are reputable scientists who still deny that link, but to say there is universal consensus is, I humbly submit, demonstrable nonsense.

There also proved to be something of another curious paradox in that the Glycemic Index Foundation are receiving up to $6000 per product from food and drink companies for a low-GI health tick.[28] Some of the products that get a tick have high levels of added sugar, including that excellent 99.4 per cent sugar Lo GI sugar.

(All up, it won't surprise you that when I interviewed Dr Barclay for the Channel Seven *Sunday Night* program, it did not end well.)

In sum, even as some of the leading members of the Dietitians Association of Australia maintain – against scant evidence and more common sense than you could jump over – that sugar consumption is falling and is not the key problem in any case, the highest diabetes councils in the land are steering those with diabetes to the Glycemic Index Foundation, who are giving the okay to foods and products loaded to the gunnels with the very substance that other reputable medical science has identified as a key cause of Type 2 diabetes in the first place!

(In the course of writing this book, I happened to be addressing 300 medical professionals – most of whom dealt with the consequences of diabetes – in an after-dinner speech. In question time, I took the liberty of asking them how many believed, in 2016, that sugar was the primary cause of Type 2 diabetes. An entire forest of hands went up around the room. And how many of you don't? Just four hands went up. When I asked the senior one of them why he said that, he maintained the cause was obesity. 'Which comes mostly from sugar?' I asked. 'Yes,' he said.)

Go figure.

Still, the pro-sugar forces continue to go hard and they don't just get help from GI fans like the aforementioned Dr Barclay and Professor Brand-Miller. Just last year one report was published which argued not just that 'Australia's sugar consumption has fallen by 16.5 per cent from 1970 to 2011, according to Australian research published in this month's *European Journal of Clinical Nutrition*', but that per capita sugar consumption peaked in Australia at 57 kilograms per year in – wait for it – 1951.[29]

Yes, if you believe the research, all of us Boomkas waddling down the street in recent years were actually having *less* sugar than those lean Aussies from 60 years ago. According to the study, Australians never consumed as much sugar as they did in 1951, back when there basically were no sugary breakfast cereals, the very year *before* Kellogg's introduced Frosties (29 per cent sugar) in 1952!

So, from the very year extra sugary cereals were introduced, sugar consumption dropped from its peak the year before?

I can smell another Paradox.

That year of the peak, 1951, was also a time, of course, before service stations also became confectionary emporiums, before the science of getting sugar into so many food and drink products became so corporately sophisticated and pervasive; before school canteens in Australia served things like soft drinks and ice-creams; before ubiquitous vending machines on every corner pumped out soft drinks and products packed with sugar; before every urban environment in the country became heavily occupied by takeaway food franchises serving up fizzy sugar-water by the tanker-load. Dr Stanton notes there were 600 to 800 food products available for sale in the 1950s and 60s and over 30,000 now. All of the above have only accelerated as phenomena as the decades have rolled on, and yet, somehow, despite all that, our sugar consumption has *fallen*? As Robertson points out, the under-appreciated issue here is that no-one is reliably measuring the consumption of added sugar in Australia. Sure, some claim to be doing so, but on closer inspection it turns out that they are doing something quite different.

The study in question, titled 'Apparent Consumption of Refined Sugar in Australia (1938-2011)', purported to show that 'Sugar consumption in Australia appears to have been relatively stable in the three decades following the end of World War 2 but since the late 1970s there has been a substantial decline.'

One of the authors of the study, Bill Shrapnel, even made the point: 'The downward trend in sugar consumption observed in our study is interesting because it runs counter to recent assumptions that sugar intake is rising and driving increasing rates of overweight and obesity in Australia. However, cause and effect conclusions cannot be drawn from our study. Given the current attention being paid to sugar, we thought it was essential that healthcare professionals and policy makers had access to recent and accurate data on trends in sugar consumption. Informed policies can now be developed from such studies.'[30]

Oh, by the way, Shrapnel works for the 'Sugar Research Advisory Service', which is funded by the sugar industry, which 'aims to provide an evidence-based view of the role of sugars in nutrition and health'.

His co-author, Tom McNeill, who formerly worked for Queensland Sugar, is a director of Greenpool Commodities, which is a consultancy employed by the sugar industry.

Interestingly, the Australian sugar series they published is based on the counting methodology that the Australian Bureau of Statistics (ABS) itself abandoned as unreliable after 1998–99. (Is this all starting to sound strangely familiar? Almost like we are wandering in a big sugary loop, rather like a donut?) Indeed, the ABS advised Rory Robertson in 2012 that its sugar series was discontinued as unreliable. That was confirmed in 2014 by ABC investigative journalist Wendy Carlisle: 'The ABS has also told [Radio National] *Background Briefing* it could no longer rely on that data because they didn't have the resources to properly count how much sugar we were eating because sugar was now embedded in our food and drink.'[31, 32]

Bill Shrapnel and Tom McNeill disagreed, and maintain that the ABS methodology they used was not broken and abandoned, but is rather a 'reliable and trusted reference for policy makers, health professionals, industry and others'.[33]

Without impugning the academic integrity of either man, can you forgive me for thinking that the dynamic which so maligned the work of John Yudkin all those decades ago – financed by the corporate power of those who sell sugar – is still alive and well in Australia in the 21st century, and it is not even restricted to those organisations specifically devoted to diet.

Let's look at the Australian Heart Foundation.

Surely, if they give a tick to a food product, you can count on it being healthy for your heart?

In a word, no.

In the case of the Australian Heart Foundation,[34] I was stunned by the observation by Gillespie that they gave the tick of approval 'to products which are sold to children which contain 70 per cent sugar', checked it out, and discovered he was right!

Look at Uncle Tobys Fruit Fix. Before it was recently withdrawn from sale after the outcry, an extraordinary 7/10ths of it was pure sugar – and yet the Australian Heart

Foundation had given it the big tick! One wonders, in passing, if a product that has 70 per cent sugar is okay with our Heart Foundation, just what percentage of sugar would have been too much for them? At what point would they withhold the tick? 80 per cent? 90 per cent?

Where exactly would they draw the line?

Does it trouble you, as it troubles me, that those companies who wish for their products to receive a tick had to first pay a 'licence fee' to the Australian Heart Foundation for the trouble of being assessed? Does it seem right to you that in so many of these health organisations, far from being removed from matters of base commerce, the money passes between the companies and the very organisation asked to give their products a clean bill of health? And that they know that if they do give it the tick, they will be able to collect an annual licence fee for as many years as that same product is on the market?

Does it trouble you, as it troubles me, that the Australian Heart Foundation is giving ticks to products loaded with the very substance that as reputable an institution as the Mayo Clinic has *specifically identified* as one that 'may pose the greatest problem for incident diabetes, diabetes-related metabolic abnormalities, and [Cardio-Vascular] risk'?[35]

I know, I know, I am merely – as one of my many critics once fabulously noted – 'a footballer who can type', but to my eyes something is seriously amiss here.

A rough equivalent would be paying *Choice* magazine to review your product, with most readers completely clueless of any money changing hands between you and the mag – and *Choice* knowing that if it does give it the thumbs-up, the money may well continue to flow for years to come.

On the specific subject of the Fruit Fix product and others like it – which are still on sale – how can this be? Sure, they are low in fat, but how could such an institution hand out ticks to food products that are just about as close to pure sugar as the human palate can handle without retching? (Particularly when, in America, Professor Gugliucci and Robert Lustig have just published a study establishing that removing such products from the diets of obese children for just nine days changes their heart risk numbers very significantly.)[36]

Did I mention that among the Australian Heart Foundation sponsors are Mackay Sugar Limited and Uncle Tobys?[37] (Which is owned by Nestlé. As you no doubt know, Nestlé has many health products like Kit Kat, Milky Bars and of course Smarties.)

Do you get that this is all part of the Big Sugar *modus operandi*? Just last year, Coca-Cola's US organisation 'fessed up to putting an extraordinary US$120 million towards such organisations as the American Academy of Pediatrics[38] (US$3m), the Academy of Family Physicians ($3.5m), the American College of Cardiology (US$3.1m), the American Cancer Society (US$2m) and the Academy of Nutrition and Dietetics (US$1.7m) as well as US$29 million sponsoring universities and *scientists* conducting academic research. What do you think they are getting for their money, if not the ability to spin their own message that their products are not all bad for health?

I contend that a lesser version of this is clearly happening in Australia.

And it is not just me or Gillespie or other anti-sugar evangelicals that are bitterly critical of this commercial relationship between the Australian Heart Foundation and those companies.

Public critics like Dr Rosemary Stanton have implied that is like 'buying a halo'.[39] 'I was critical because people had to pay for it,' she said, '[whereas] it was always described as "we earned the tick", as if you were selected.'

The good news is that the Australian Heart Foundation seems to have at least partly seen the light, and announced in December 2015 that they would be stopping the program in due course, while noting, 'The Heart Foundation will continue to work with manufacturers who currently have the Tick on their products as the program winds down. It is expected the program will be fully retired over the next 12 to 24 months.'[40] I am hoping 'fully retired' means 'taken out the back and shot'. If so, bravo.

But while the American Heart Association – which has no such sponsors – has a firm guideline that no woman should have more than six teaspoons of sugar a day and no man more than nine teaspoons, our own Australian Heart Foundation still has no such limit. They claim to be okay if a quarter of our daily calories come from sugar, which is to say 21 teaspoons!

At least the Australian Competition and Consumer Commission gives a bugger, and recently hauled Heinz[41] over the coals for marketing its toddler food Shredz as

'99 per cent fruit and veg' and therefore the best way to get those toddlers aged one to three years old to 'independently discover the delicious taste of nutritious food' and 'inspire a love of nutritious food that lasts a lifetime'.

What was the problem?

Try this: the snack is more than 60 per cent sugar!

'If you look at something saying it's "99 per cent fruit and veg" which it prominently displayed,' ACCC chairman Rod Sims was quoted as saying, 'most people would think that's fairly low in sugar.'

Yup. And of course junior wolfs it down, just as humans have instinctively done since the dawn of time, on those rare occasions when fresh fruit comes their way. When better to fill the reserve tank? The problem comes in the modern age, when parents who don't realise what they're doing are filling junior's reserve tank all day, every day!

Meanwhile, in August 2016, just as this manuscript goes off to the publisher, the American Heart Association released a scientific statement recommending that 'added sugars should not be included *at all* in the diet of children under the age of 2 years'.[42] Things are moving. At least over there . . .

Here in Australia, though, there are still no such recommendations.

It is, my friends, a *scandal*.

What I do say is this, and I mean it:

There continues to be a war going on out there over the effect of our diet on our health and weight, much the same one that's been going on since the days of Keys and Yudkin.

It is for the hearts and minds and, most particularly, the bellies of the people. (Though, interestingly, as most of the Keys/Yudkin battle was in the 50s and 60s, most of their battle was around heart disease rather than weight, for the simple reason that obesity was so much less common, and not really a community problem. Dr Rosemary Stanton comments that when she did her first school canteen survey in 1967, 'We were concerned about sugar, but because of its effect on teeth. Obese kids were so rare that weight didn't figure!')

Now, on one side is a large chunk of the food and drink industry which makes *billions* of dollars by selling products completely rotten with sugar, which inevitably makes those bellies get ever larger. On the other side are the growing band of doctors, independent nutrition experts and know-nothing-but-suddenly-slimmer-loudmouths like me, who actually realise the truth and say it out loud – it bloody well *is* sugar which is making everyone obese and we would all be better off cutting our sugar intake back to the bone.

I agree with Lustig, who says, 'Politicians have to come in and reset the playing field, as they have with any substance that is toxic and abused, ubiquitous and with negative consequence for society. Alcohol, cigarettes . . . We don't have to ban any of them. We don't have to ban sugar. But the food industry cannot be given *carte blanche*. They're allowed to make money, but they're not allowed to make money by making people sick.'[43]

And this is far from merely an Australian problem. In America, their DAA equivalent, the Academy of Nutrition and Dietetics, has Coke, Pepsi and Kellogg's among their sponsors.[44] Their rivals, the American Society for Nutrition, has all of the above, plus McDonald's and Nestlé.[45] The British Nutrition Foundation, meanwhile, gets funding from Nestlé, Kellogg's, PepsiCo and Coca-Cola.[46] The Dietitians of Canada association has 'partnerships' with McDonald's, Coca-Cola, Nestlé and PepsiCo.[47]

And we wonder why obesity levels in all these countries are soaring?

My solution?

I thought you'd never ask!

It is two-fold. In Australia, the Federal Government should do its bit to fund such organisations as the Dietitians Association of Australia[48] and the Australian Heart Foundation, as well as providing proper funding for research in the field.

In the case of the DAA, it is singularly important. If a dietitian wishes to get a job with the government in any capacity, or for their patients to get refunds from health funds, then they must be accredited with the DAA – giving them enormous official clout. So doesn't it make sense that such an important body as the DAA receive government funding, to liberate it from the need to have any relationship whatsoever with Big Sugar?

In the words of Professor Stephen Simpson of Sydney University, who works in the field, 'We need to free academia and the medical foundations from having to take money from industry.' His idea is to have some kind of Industry Future Fund, whereby all food and beverage industries contribute to a fund that is then administered independently by the Federal Government.

And, yes, I know it would be interesting to see just how quick the food and beverage companies would be to hand over money to such an organisation once their influence could not be so directly applied, but still . . .

I think it would be worth it for the government to provide the money just for the benefits to the health of the population alone. The money would easily be made up by the savings made on the taxpayer from having to pay ever larger hospital bills for a population getting ever bigger.

Professor Alejandro Gugliucci, who has worked and lectured in France, Canada, Uruguay, Japan and US, agrees that the key is to liberate such organisations from the corporate teat, noting of Big Sugar, 'They have tons of lawyers and scientists literally on their payroll to bring down Rob Lustig, me and our team and all the others by biased science and/or character assassination. [Still,] as Gandhi said: "First they ignore you, next they laugh at you. Then they attack you and then you win." We are now at the third stage . . .'

Canada recently went through the process of getting funding for such organisations, and the results were remarkable. As documented by Gillespie, the Canadian Heart and Stroke Foundation also had a record of 'plumbing new lows in prostituting health advice to the interests of the food industry',[49] which, in their case, included taking money to give a 'Check' of approval to Slush Puppies, with six and a half teaspoons of sugar in it and gave the same tick to the Sunrype Fruitsource Bites that was 80 per cent sugar by weight and 96 per cent by calories! And yet, in 2014, shortly after they weaned themselves off corporate money, they did a rapid about-turn and came out strongly against sugar, noting in a public statement that 'excess sugar consumption is associated with adverse health effects including heart disease, stroke, obesity, diabetes, high blood cholesterol, cancer and dental cavities . . .'. And this was merely its opening remarks!

'In a single document they have catapulted themselves from handmaiden of the processed food industry to the world leader in health policy.'[50]

Surely, it is obvious we should do the same in Australia?

In the meantime, as a bare beginning, why not put on the front of every article of processed food and every can and bottle of processed drink unit sold, a clear number to indicate just how many teaspoons of sugar are in it? Wouldn't most sane people think twice before reaching for a can of Coke if it had emblazoned on it the words nine teaspoons of sugar? Peters choc-mint drumstick – five teaspoons of sugar. Forty gram Crunchie bar – just under seven teaspoons of sugar.

And Australia should impose a sugar tax, too, just as Britain has recently introduced, following the lead of Mexico.

A pause here, while the critics cry out, 'Nanny state! Nanny state!'

Now that would be fine if you critics weren't wanting that same Nanna to look after you when you are crook and in hospital with so many ailments brought on by overconsumption of sugar!

All I'm saying is that if you insist on pouring sugar down your gullet now, isn't it fair that you start to pay your inevitable hospital bills now, just as the tobacco tax helps to pay for the cancer wards? Who better to pay the costs of ill-health than those choosing to live unhealthily? And just as the tobacco tax and tobacco education campaigns have been successful over the years – taking the number of Australians smoking down from 75 per cent in the 1950s to about 13 per cent now – making our lungs healthier because of it,[51] so too can sugar tax and education be equally effective.

In the meantime, the struggle over public health policy goes on.

Now, we all know what the tobacco industry did when confronted with the growing realisation among the medical establishment and then the government and finally the people, that smoking caused cancer. The head honchos – seeing what the coming reduction in smoking would do to their profits – organised a calculated campaign of obfuscation, which included putting heavy funding behind any scientist they could find who would write reports, give lectures and say in the media that smoking caused no harm. At the very least, they had to delay action being taken, so their profits could go on for as long as possible. And they were devastatingly effective.

As late as 1996 in the US, the Republican Presidential candidate Bob Dole was saying to a stunned Katie Couric on the *Today Show* that smoking wasn't that bad and that drinking milk was potentially as harmful to your heart and

133

health as smoking. No, *really*. And he wasn't being sneaky. Dole genuinely believed it. And he was amazed when all the sane people in America said, 'I'm sorry, what was that crap you just said?'

This was because he had spent his life smoking, while also being told for much of it by respectable paid experts and lobbyists that smoking was not really that bad, not if you did it in moderation.

Of course, a lot of smokers are not moderate, they tend to be addicted, just like people are addicted to sugar. But back in the 1950s it was only the real health kooks that suggested that you should stop smoking. And that was only if you were pregnant.

Does anyone see a pattern of behaviour here? Is a flashing light going off? Apart from the one as you open and close the fridge door, I mean?

The fossil fuel industry is doing exactly the same now, before our very eyes, trying to delay action on climate change. They're making billions, and nothing can be allowed to get in the way of that, particularly nothing that will curb those profits.

Yes, the overwhelming evidence from objective science clearly points to a future disaster – that is preventable if we act now – but why pay attention to that when we have paid contrarians at the ready, happy to distract you with alternative facts and reassuring dubious theories? Nothing to see here, the science is not in, the debate continues, everyone just keep doing exactly what you are doing, no need to change your behaviour or our profit margin.

So, bearing all that in mind, what are the chances that the sugar industry, with *billions* of dollars at stake, isn't doing something similar to defend itself?

And why, exactly, would companies manufacturing sugary products be sponsoring something like the Dietitians Association of Australia and the Australian Heart Foundation? Do you *really* think it's just because they want to get the message out there that everyone should be eating healthily?

What's in it for them? What is the return you think they're getting for the millions of dollars they're putting in? If it was me, and my sponsorship/partnership dollars, I would want to be bloody sure that everything coming out of those associations, and all articles written and statements made by people connected to them, *didn't* make people want to cut their sugar intake.

Plus, it's a nice look for Big Sugar – they are not trying to make you fat with sugar, they are interested in your nutrition and your heart. After all, they give money to the Dietitians Association of Australia and the Heart Foundation! I rest my case and put away all thoughts of a class action mass obesity lawsuit, Your Honour.

Still, maybe their defenders are right, and maybe it's all ridgy-didge, rinky-dink, and true-blue. Maybe it is fine that the sugar companies sponsor the health organisations.

Or . . . maybe not.

Still, think on this:

Twenty-five years ago, when I was putting together a book called *Little Theories of Life*, a reader drew to my attention that 'after any tragedy, accident, disaster, siege or disturbance, or just about any newsworthy incident what-soever . . . the eye-witnesses always start off their accounts with "*Well, first I heard a bang . . .*"'

And they were right! Ever since, watching the news, I always pause when they get to the first eye-witness account.

'Well, first I heard a bang . . .'

Every time.

So, now that I have clued you up a little, take a look at the next news story purporting to give you the good oil on how to lose weight – often attached to a just released report or survey to give it a news 'hook'. Now see how often the upshot of the story, subtle or otherwise, is that it really is okay to consume sugar, and those of us who waffle on about the dangers of it should just eat waffles soaked with syrup as they do, and there is no problem.

It is not about sugar they say. It is portion size! (Which would be fine, if the sugar didn't make you want ever larger portions.)

Or . . . sugar is fine, they say. The true problem is, when you replace the sugar snacks with something else, like chips, it's worse. (So stick with sugar snacks!) Oh, and let's not forget the Easter staple: chocolate. (It is actually good for you, don't you know?)

Best of all, even sugar in processed food is a 'natural product' and as long as you take it in moderation, no problem. (But few readers of this book have matched that description over the years, I would suggest. It seems to me that dieticians who say this are like traffic cops telling motorists not to speed, too often . . . like an oncologist noting that one or two cigarettes a day are much less likely to kill you than a pack a day. Like the little thing at the end of the long gambling ad, telling you to gamble responsibly.)

It's amazing how many such stories there are out there, and how aware of them you become, once you are clued up as to what is going on.

Lustig, in his seminal lecture, sets out how exactly the same dynamic is at work in America, though he notes that in their case, the Federal bodies meant to regulate food and drink consumption are doing no such thing.

'So the [Food and Drug Administration] isn't touching this,' he says, referring to the infestation of what he calls a *poison*, fructose, through so much, and so many, of America's food and drink products. 'The US [Department of Agriculture] isn't touching this, because if the USDA touched this, what would that mean? That would mean an admission to the world that our food is a problem. So what do you think that would do . . .? So the USDA doesn't want to know about this, because this is bad news. And so who runs the food pyramid? The USDA – it's the fox in charge of the henhouse, because their job is to sell food. And who is eating it? We are.'[52]

And we in Australia are, too.

If you can see this as clearly as I do, it will make you doubly determined to slim down, as your own body will be the best advertisement possible in helping to lead our whole population back to health.

And yes, seeing as you ask, I *do* expect this book to take flak from that broad lobby, just as David Gillespie, Robert Lustig,

Professor Alejandro Gugliucci and Sarah Wilson, author of the *I Quit Sugar* series, and all the rest have come under fire, as the sugar lobby tries to poke holes in their credentials or lack thereof, and more particularly their science.

Well, they're in for a nice surprise when they try to attack *my* credentials.

See, I don't have *any*! Attack *that*, you mongrels!

And then explain, perhaps, why – when the solution is so damn simple – your every utterance has not been to put that solution, STOP THE SUGAR, front and centre!

Meantime, what I can point to is that I have lost 45 kilos by getting my head around the basic principles that the anti-sugar brigade espouse, and embracing those principles in my selection of what I do and don't put in my mouth.

The net consequence for you readers is that if you – like me – radically cut your sugar intake, there are five obvious outcomes that are simply beyond dispute.

First, your level of hunger will drop.

Second, you will eat less.

Third, with fewer calories coming in through sugar, and less food overall, you will lose weight.

Fourth, you are likely to have a healthier liver, prevent diabetes and heart attacks.

Fifth, and most importantly, you will be healthier!

And the problem would be what, exactly, Officer? What is not to like about all those outcomes?

And as to all the hand-wringing over the idea that by demonising sugar we give a free pass to all the other baddies out there – palm oil being a notable example, together with trans fats, lack of fibre, etc – I call bullshit. For starters, if you avoid sugar by steering away from processed foods, the other baddies disappear too, as they are found in the same products. And remember Lustig's earlier point. It is not as if we need any sugar. If people don't get their sugar hit, the body doesn't even blink.

Dr Rosemary Stanton has been warning of the dangers of sugar throughout her 50-year career and notes to me that, 'cutting out sugar also cuts out a lot of the other junk found in foods that contain sugar – such as cakes, biscuits, pastries, confectionery and many desserts. This all results in a reduction in kilojoules.'

And I repeat. It is not just that the sugar is bad for you in its own right, it is that it stuffs up the rest of your system, and continues to make you want more. If this was the Dietary Wild West, who can doubt that sugar would be top of the pops on the Most Wanted posters with a $500 reward on its head? It is not just another food group, it is the ingredient that stuffs up your entire system.

There are, nevertheless, a couple of areas where I respectfully differ from Gillespie, whose book first sent me down this path.

It's not quite that he gives a free pass to wine and other alcoholic beverages, it's just that I sort of read it that way.

'Most alcoholic drinks,' he wrote in *Sweet Poison*, 'do not contain significant amounts of fructose, it being one of the sugars fermented to create the alcohol. Beer contains lots of maltose but is fructose free. Most wines are largely fructose free . . . Most hard liquor is also fructose free, as long as you don't add mixers (besides water) to them.'

The upshot was that even while I embarked on cutting out sugar, I continued to guzzle wine like a mad thing. It would take me a little more time to get my head around that crucial part of this Great Aussie Bloke Slim-Down equation, too. For that, please do read on . . .

EIGHT

Giving up the grog

'It was my Uncle George who discovered that alcohol was a food well in advance of modern medical thought . . .'
P. G. Wodehouse, author and humorist

'I got sober. I stopped killing myself with alcohol. I began to think: "Wait a minute – if I can stop doing this, what are the possibilities?" And slowly it dawned on me that it was maybe worth the risk . . .'
Craig Ferguson, Scottish comedian

'One more drink, and I would have been under the host . . .'
Dorothy Parker, writer and satirist

I already know what you're thinking, just from reading the chapter title. You are thinking that whatever happens, you will wait till hell freezes over, pigs fly past a blue moon, and Pauline Hanson is prime minister before you ever try *that* solution.

But I am here to tell you, it dinkum is possible, and a better life awaits. My name is Peter and – strangely, given how much I was drinking – I am not an alcoholic. But I was overweight and the grog was not helping. In fact, alcohol was the enabler-in-chief, liquid permission to eat whatever I liked – and what I never realised until recently was the damage the grog was doing to me *in calories alone.*

Let me tell you my story, first up.

Outside of football tours and 21st birthday parties, I was never much of a heavy drinker until about ten years ago when, under a huge amount of pressure – doing breakfast radio, while meeting book deadlines and raising three teenagers with a wife who had just started anchoring breakfast television – I would knock back a bottle of wine, if not two, most days. My basic reasoning was that there was no problem in the world so great that one good bottle of chardonnay couldn't solve it – in the short term – and with two bottles of wine over lunch and dinner, I could feel confident and happy, like my old self, if even only for a few hours. Before I knew it I was drinking heavily and not just liking it, but loving it!

I repeat, I was not an alcoholic, at least not by Australian standards, but by gawd on a bad day I reckon I could have held my own with one. But then came my next epiphany.

On 14 September 2014, I had driven all day from Sydney down to Thredbo to pick up my second son after he had completed a three-month stint as a ski instructor, and I was having dinner with my mate Jordan Rodgers, who runs the whole shebang.

I had polished off the first bottle of wine after 20 minutes, as you do, and had sent up an emergency distress flare for the waitress to please quickly bring me another, when I said to my mate, more than a little curiously, 'You're not drinking, Jordan . . . ?'

Now, as you know, the translation for this in Aussie-bloke-speak is very simple: 'Call yourself my mate, an Australian male, we're catching up on a Friday night, and you're not on your way to being pissed as a newt, just like me? What is WRONG with you?'

'No,' Jordan said. 'I guess, running Thredbo, I feel I should bring my A-game to it. On a busy day we have 7000 people here and it is a fair responsibility.'

Bingo!

I thought about it deeply while guzzling my way through the next bottle.

The next day, I tried to ski with my lad, Louis.

Now, as you know, dear reader, for fatties like us there is a very fine line between what others call 'skiing' and what you and I might call 'trying to get the fuck off the mountain as quickly as possible!' The fate of Sonny Bono haunts many a large man as he whistles downwards towards the danger-ously still trees. (And I don't just mean marrying Cher.)

I mean, snow, gravity, weight and alcohol are not a safe combination and, danger aside, it is just hideously uncomfortable.

I came down, feeling old, fat and slow – and all the moreso for being right next to my young, fit and athletic son, the very man I used to be, only three short decades ago. The chilly wind whistled off the mountain.

Ah, sing it with me! *I pulled my harpoon out of my dirty red bandana, I was playing soft, while Bobby sang the blues, yeah . . .*

Of course, I did the obvious. As a matter of fact, I did what you and I have *always* done whenever feeling a tad low and a lot slow. I had a huge meal that night and got maggoted! Distress flares were going off all over the restaurant.

We need more wine to Table 5 on the double! Because that's the way we roll, am I right?

On and on, into the dark and stormy night.

Windshield wipers slapping time, I was holding Bobby's hand in mine, we sang every song that driver knew . . .

Still, the seed of the previous evening had taken root, and by the time I woke, on that Sunday morning, coming down – feeling near as faded as my jeans – something was different. Sure, I was foggy, slow and seedy as per usual, but this time I was so physically rooted as well from the excess of exercise the previous day that I really focused on the possibility of doing something different . . .

Why not, like Jordan, try stopping grog altogether? Just the way I had stopped smoking? And sugar in food, soft drinks and fruit juices? And coffee? Where better to start going cold turkey than Thredbo on a freezing, windy day?

In fact, not drinking that Sunday during the day was easy, as I was driving back to Sydney, sneering unpleasantly at the Goulburn McDonald's as I passed. But that evening, instead of defiantly opening a wine over dinner with Lisa – yes, my love, stare, I don't care (*pop*) – I skipped it. She noted it, but said nothing.

Strangely, I didn't miss it a bit, and woke the next morning with – hold the phones and snuggle in tight, my love – a totally clear head.

That week I went to several lunches and a dinner where again, oddly, I just felt virtuous, as those around me started slurring their words in, let's face it, a most pathetic fashion. (*Please tell me I didn't used to carry on like that, did I? I did? Well, sorry.*) Even more interesting, one of the lunches and one of the dinners were corporate affairs where I was the guest speaker and, if I do say so myself, I was able to nail both of them as never before. It's not that I ever did corporate speeches drunk, but I now realised that even with two wines in me, I had limited my ability to read the room, to time the anecdotes, to work out what to say next. Stone-cold sober, everything worked, and I could get it pitch-perfect.

The best thing of all?

On that next Saturday morning, I checked my weight, and found that I had gone down two kilograms!

On Saturday night, it was my eldest lad's 21st birthday party and after one more sober speech, I lifted the glass, filled with champagne.

'Here's to Jake,' I cried cheerily, as the song-throng all joined me in the toast.

But this was the moment, and I somehow knew it. (And you will know it, mate. Because you and I are cut from the same cloth.) If I had just one sip, it would have been *ridic-ulous* – weak, wan, wanker-ish – not to have two sips. Who *does* that? And this *was* my beautiful first-born boy's 21st!

Against that, I knew the drill as well as I know myself. If I could have two sips, why not four? Why not the whole glass? Of course it wouldn't hurt to have two glasses, because if one glass of grog is nice, two glasses are great, a whole bottle is fabulous, and with two bottles in me, I always had the time of my life. At least I think I did, if only I could remember any of it.

But it all goes by in a bit of a blur, doesn't it, mate?

So on this Saturday night, at this key moment when the weakness was starting to take hold and crush me, instead of buckling, I resisted. Didn't even have a single sip. And I haven't had a sip of grog since. And I won't, until the night Australia grows up and becomes a republic, but that's another story. (And another book, come to think of it. Still, Her Majesty always seems to be in terrific shape, while Queen Victoria . . . not so much.)

The upside of this stopping grog completely? Let me count the ways!

1. **Mate, no joke, the weight just FALLS off you.** Each bottle of wine – and this was a revelation to me – has more calories than a Big Mac![1] Who knew? I certainly didn't. How many times have I had a three-course lunch at a fancy restaurant, washed down by a couple of Big Macs, gone home for dinner, and then wondered why I had turned into a Fatty Boomka? If beer is your poison,

work off the notion that it only takes four cans of beer to equal a Big Mac.

2. **You really do bring your A-game to everything.** You think clearly, need less sleep, and are twice as productive. Without alcohol in me, I can focus for sustained periods and do much higher quality work. In my own field of writing, I have often finished writing something while pissed, certain that it was Pulitzer-bait, only to read it sober the next morning and realise it is tragic trash. I sometimes wonder if architects get caught in the same syndrome, and *that* is the explanation for some of the more outlandish buildings you see across our brown and pleasant land. But enough about Federation Square . . .

3. **You have so much more money.** For starters, restaurant bills are about half. Oh, and the ill-disciplined drunk-spend – that surge of what-the-hell-I'll-buy-the-bastard – disappears!

4. **Your willpower is so much stronger, across the board.** We all know the phenomenon of blokes giving up smoking, right up until Saturday night when – drunk as a skunk in a cellar – they reach for a bunger and are back on them again. For me that was less of a problem than having too much grog in me when a plate of party pies went by!

You remember Edward Scissorhands? Well, with a plate of *hors d'oeuvres* within cooee, I used to turn into Peter Hoover-Hands. I could simply move my hands over the plate and all those scrumptious little things would be sucked up into my vortex, in about six seconds flat. Waiters and waitresses used to line up before me, knowing I was the easiest way to head back to the kitchen with an empty plate without the hassle of having to circulate. But stone-cold sober, I can stop myself!

5. **You get it through your thick noggin, at last: while it is a better night with grog, it is a better life without.** And it really is. And when you get to the end of a week, it really is more than a blur of drink-fests with dull parts in between, when you are waiting for the next drink-fest. (Somewhere or other I came across a quote from the famed American writer and alcoholic Caroline Knapp: 'When you quit drinking, you stop waiting . . .'[2] Doesn't that make you shift uncomfortably?)

6. **You sleep better.** I have never understood all that mumbo-jumbo about REM deep-sleep patterns and all that gibberish, but I can tell you this. After years of going to bed with a bellyful of grog, only to get up several times during the night, the chance of uninter-rupted sleep was a revelation. And the best thing is . . .

7. **You wake up, ready to rock and roll!** For years, I would get out of bed feeling, as the saying goes, as if someone had left the Dead Sea Scrolls in my mouth overnight for safe-keeping. You, too? Well, let's face it: we did that so often, that became the *normal* feeling upon waking. But no more! How good is it to wake up early, get moving and hit the day, unburdened by lethargy, headaches, a furry mouth or grouchiness.

8. **That feeling of wellbeing gets stronger as each day goes on.** You will likely remember the immortal words of Dean Martin, who was in a position to know. 'I feel sorry for people who don't drink. Because when they wake up, that's as good as they are going to feel for the whole damn day.' Simply not true. Just having the energy to do so many things changes everything.

9. **Any other addictions you might have – be they cigarettes, chocolate bars or (heaven forbid) the pokies – will become easier to deal with.** Your willpower will be stronger, and you will feel more in control than you ever have. It's easy to say no to something you know is bad for you or dangerous to your wellbeing – and yes, Boomka, I *do* mean Cheryl from Accounts, too – when you're stone-cold sober and thinking clearly.

10. **Brownie points! Happy wife, happy life.** Even when Lisa is pissed off at me for something – mostly being a lazy slob around the house, seeing as you ask – I have so many Brownie points in the kitty for being 45 kilos lighter than I was, and 100 per cent sober all the time, and more pleasant to be with, that we get through it quickly. For me, beyond health, this last one is the biggest plus to the whole thing. So let's go into it a little bit deeper . . .

See, Boomka, for the moment I will leave you and your relationship out of this and talk about mine. It's a good one! We met on 7 December 1991, were engaged three months later, married another six months on, and have been together ever after.

But it's not a Hallmark greeting card relationship, it's a real one.

By my reckoning, over that time, we've had on average 300 pretty good days together a year, 50 fabulous days and . . . 15 *shockers*.

What causes the shockers? Broadly, I would say, like everyone, it comes down to the struggle to juggle. When you have too many things on, too little time to get through them, balls are dropped. Whose fault are those dropped balls?

Well, when pissed, I not only would have said they were *her* fault, but frequently *did* say so!

Sometimes loudly.

Now . . . not so much.

Without grog in you, you are much less often a bad-tempered prick, and I really mean that. I am not a moody bastard by nature, and was lucky that when I had too much grog in me, the primary effect was to make me more inclined to laugh, or lie down for a sleep. Yet there really was another side to it, looking back. I never used to think grog could affect my temper, but, on sober reflection, it did.

For starters, when I am sober, I am no longer inclined to tell my wife, *wit' shum detail, now you lishen to me* . . . a few things she DESPERATELY needed to be told at the time!

Why bother? With sobriety, I am juggling better and dropping far fewer balls. I have more energy for her and our children, I am calmer, and when things do go wrong, as they inevitably will, I am much less likely to blow up in frustration.

Bottom line?

At the very least, at the bare, hungry, sniffin' MINIMUM, you should give giving up the grog entirely a try. Go for a week, for starters, and see how you go. It might amaze you, seriously, how not being pissed is a piece of piss, precisely because not being pissed is after all our natural state. Your body will thank you for it, not to mention your partner. I will warm to the virtues of total abstinence in a later chapter, but for now try it, like I did. Not moderation, just . . . stop.

And, yes, of course I accept that it will be difficult for many people, and an agony for alcoholics. I genuinely feel for you. But the pity of it is, there must be hundreds of thousands of blokes from Penrith to Perth, Darwin to the Derwent, and particularly north of the Tweed who – just like me – could give it up without too much trouble, and live a different, better life, but have never even tried. Since I wrote that initial column in the *Herald* I have been overwhelmed by fabulous – and in many instances, quite emotional – letters from blokes who have noted how, like me, they only wish they had done it years ago. They've dropped the pud, lifted their energy levels, repaired their relationships, saved heaps of money and are more productive than ever in their work. I repeat: what's not to like?

Of course, if you lay off the grog, you'll get grilled. I certainly did. But arm yourself with forethought and a good response, and you'll be fine, mate. Here are a few of the more poetic questions I was asked.

FAQ. Are you out of your fucking mind?

This is a serious question, heard most often from blokes you've known for 30 years. See, you and I have knocked about together at lunches, long afternoons and dinners over that time, been on football trips, and between us we've drunk enough to float a battleship and now you don't want to drink anymore? What is wrong with you? My answer is, stop slobbering all over me, you drunken bum! And, more seriously, I gently encourage mates to try it, and not to knock it until they have done so.

FAQ. Are you a wanker?

No. Are you? Plenty of people drink happily in moderation, and good luck to them. It's only when I stopped drinking, however, I could see clearly so much of the devastation wrought by the heavy drinking that is ingrained in Australian life. In a way I never could before, I could see how many broken marriages, strained relationships, familial fractures, lost jobs and myriad messes were caused, one way or another, by blokes getting so regularly on the piss that it became a staple of their lives without them even realising. And that's not even counting the DUIs, the impulsive decisions taken while under the influence that end up ruining whole lives – including those of their loved ones. And in my experience it is mostly those heavy drinkers that give you the hardest time about not drinking yourself.

FAQ. Why don't you have just one drink, it won't kill you?

I hear this one all the time – or at least I used to, for the first six months. It is the pressure to rejoin the pack, be one of the boys, knock it back, get it into yer! And oddly for one who has drunk as much as I have, I am not remotely tempted. It wasn't that the old life was bad. Far from it. But this one is better.

FAQ. Do you lose all your drinking mates?

It's been amazing to me how often I'm asked that. And the short answer is, yes, a bit. My wise brother Andrew once noted to me that 'singles move with singles, couples hang with couples, married couples with married couples, and married couples with children hang with married couples with children', and exactly the same applies to big drinkers. Personally, when I was on the grog, loving it, I would naturally gravitate to events where plenty of grog was a part of the occasion, and that would include lunches and dinners with big-drinking mates. I still love 'em as much as ever, and I think they do me the same honour but, truthfully, I really don't see as much of them as I did. Against that, nor am I hanging out more with the local Temperance Society of Tee-Totalling Turkeys. I guess I'm just working harder, putting a lot more energy and time into my other passions, and spending more time with my family. Be careful, this happiness could happen to you. I told you, it is a different life. A mate of both Jordan's and mine, Henry, who got off the grog before me, gave me a tip which I have found to be right on the money: 'You laugh less, but when you do, it is more genuine.'

Bottom line? If all you had in common was alcohol, then you probably didn't lose a great mate.

FAQ. When you are at a lunch or dinner, do you really sit there and drink water?

Nuh. Personally, I could now drink tea for Australia. You will work it out, but tea is what does it for me. I love it and I drink it every bit as much to excess, and more, as I used to knock back alcohol. My polite request to waiters and waitresses at restaurants is, 'Please bring me more tea than you think is good for me.'

It gives me something to do with my hands at lunches and dinners – and means that I am sipping when everyone else is sipping.

FAQ. What else changes in your life?

You actively WANT to be pulled over by the cops for a breath test! I'd like to think that in my truly adult life in Australia I have never been over the limit while behind the wheel, but there really have been times when I've seen blue flashing lights up ahead and my stomach muscles have clenched, as I work out just how long ago I'd had my last drink, how many I'd had, and just what my blood alcohol level would be now. One time, I was way too close for comfort, and came in at .04! Oh, the horror. These days, I really do actively hope to be pulled over. Pick me, Officer, pick ME! Everything is so much simpler now.

Especially getting home. There have been more than a few times, just to be on the safe side, I've taken a circuitous route back to my front door, trying to avoid the most likely places the breathalyser might wait for me. Many Australian men play out this semi-alcoholic stealth version of *Hogan's Heroes* every weekend.

We all make mistakes, but the last place you want to make one is behind the wheel of a two-tonne death machine. Cut alcohol out of the equation and you'll be much less likely to make a fatal mistake.

Cut it out, lads, wave to the cops as you drive by – or smile like you've won the lottery when they stop you.

FAQ. Any motivational tips on how I can do it?

Yes, you've come to the right place! Oddly enough, the best line of all, in terms of the reasons to stop drinking, came from my eldest son, Jake: 'When you drink, you are just borrowing fun from tomorrow.'

Bingo. I recognised the truth. Of course it is huge fun for a few hours on a Saturday night, but don't you pay for it all Sunday? Don't you come out behind on the deal? And, as I noted before, doesn't it all go by in a blur when you drink every day? *Stop*, you bastard! At least give stopping a go. What do you have to lose? If you're one of the lucky ones, as I turned out to be, it will be dead easy and your only regret will be that you didn't do it years ago and . . .

And what? You don't think outright stopping altogether is your go, and that you can just restrict your intake, and still blow out on the odd Saturday night?

You mean, just like you've tried for the last 30 years?

Okay, well, if you say so. I mean, if you really think it is going to work this time, the way it didn't work the last thousand times? You mean the way it worked when you tried to give up smoking, in exactly the same manner, until you came to the sad realisation that the only way was to stop being a chicken and actually reach out for the cold turkey?

Okay, if you say so. Sounds unlikely to me. Because if you and I were made like that, and truly understood the virtues of moderation over abstinence, how would we ever have got ourselves into the situation where we could hold our own with a baby hippo on the other end of the seesaw?

Maybe read the next chapter with a view to changing your approach?

NINE

The virtues of abstinence

'Abstinence is the great strengthener and clearer of reason . . .'
Robert South, 17th-century English preacher

'An ounce of prevention is worth a pound of cure . . .'
Benjamin Franklin

'Better to sleep with a sober cannibal than a drunk Christian . . .'
from *Moby Dick* by Herman Melville

In the early hours of 4 July 1918, General John Monash unveiled his master battle plan at Le Hamel on the Somme, a legendary clash that would come to define his career as the best General on either side of the First World War.

For four years the Allies had been trying to crack the German line on the Western Front – which stretched for 700 kilometres from the English Channel to Switzer-land – using everything from waves of soldiers, to tanks, to intense artillery on specific points, to planes bombing the bejesus out of their trenches, only to suffer horrendous losses and achieve minimal success. The genius of Monash – who once said the most impressive man he ever met was Ned Kelly, but I digress – was to come up with one coherent plan with precise down-to-the-second moves that all of the Australians involved understood, and followed to the letter. Tanks provided the spearhead and cover for the troops, who went forward as ever before, but this time in darkness, after dummy attacks to throw the German defences off. Minutely coordinated creeping artillery fire kept the German heads down at the precise instant it was necessary. And though bombers had been used before, this time Monash got the oldest, noisiest ones available to fly as low as possible, so under the cover of that sound, the tanks could be moved forward, as close as possible before the Germans became aware of them. Other bombers were later used during the attack, not to bomb the enemy, but to resupply the infantry with more ammunition and grenades.

Like a superb conductor of a great orchestra, Monash was able to coordinate his men and his weaponry in such a manner as had never been done before, and the result was a military triumph, like they just don't make 'em anymore. The Australians broke through, the Germans fell back in disarray, Monash's model was embraced by other Allied armies and the war was over just a little over four months later. It wasn't that Monash had come up with a new weapon, or fresh troops, it was that he worked out exactly the right formula to achieve maximum impact, not just on that night, but for the rest of the campaign.

Frankly, I feel much the same about the approach I have taken to getting healthy. For yonks I have known about the basic tools to do it – eating and drinking less, not eating too much food, exercising more – but it is only recently that I worked out how to synthesise them into one coherent plan. And while it has been obvious to others for yonks, it bloody well hasn't been obvious to me.

But the true breakthrough, the thing that brings them all together?

It was coming to understand that the way I am made, the approach I take to life and my passion for it, could be a liability if I took the same approach to eating and drinking. So I had to take exactly that same approach – because I can't change it – and apply it to health. And I suspect you are the same.

Let me explain.

One Friday night, when I was maybe ten years old, Mum and I were watching a movie at home in our farmhouse at Peats Ridge. It was well past my bedtime, but Mum let me stay up, 'cos it was such a strong movie. The climactic moment comes when an old man makes a forceful speech to a young woman who has been so unhappy she has even contemplated ending her own life. The old man puts a gentle hand on her shoulder and lets her have it.

'Marian,' he says, 'don't you realise? You have within you the wonder of the force of life, the same force that makes the flowers bloom, the trees grow tall, the birds to sing and the lion to roar. This force of life is a precious, precious thing and you must not waste a moment of it! You must suck the juice from the marrow of life and let it run down your chin!'

I look at Mum. Mum looks at me. That's the way I want to live. Not pretty, not neat, but passionate.

And it is the way I have lived ever since. And it has been the right way – for me. And I'll bet for you, mate?

I actually think heaps of blokes who got as big as us lived that way because the careful way, the moderate way, the sensible and careful way of eating was just anathema to us. It was not in our nature. And it is *still* not in our nature.

The answer?

What has worked for me is to accept that while a moderate approach to what you eat and drink is admirable and sensible – it just doesn't work for me.

It would be great for me if, going into every meal, I could sensibly pick and choose what I am going to eat and drink, and work out just how much grog and ice-cream etc. But I can't live like that, and frankly don't want any of my head-space going to that kind of stuff every time I sit down for a meal.

As mentioned earlier, since walking Kokoda in 2002, I haven't smoked a cigarette, or even had a drag on one.

And it was at Thredbo that I came to exactly the same conclusion about grog. I had tried moderation. It just doesn't do it for me. Moderation works for moderate people. I'm not one of them. I reckon I could make the case that, almost by definition, all badly overweight people are not moderate by nature. Do not think you will change the type of person you are. (Maybe ask your wife how she went on that project?) Instead, harness the type of person you are. Somewhere in me, for whatever reason, is the hardwired notion that if one piece of cake is good, then two pieces of cake is twice as good, just as three pieces is fabulous. And if you think you had a good time with a mate over a bottle of wine as you celebrated the anniversary of the World Cup win, WE had an even greater time over several bottles of wine!

I know, I know . . . ludicrous, and embarrassing to say out loud. But such is the way of many of us.

See, it's just in there, in my soul, no matter how much my intellect tells me that such an approach is nonsensical. And while I know those suffering anorexia have equally intellectually unsustainable beliefs in their own soul that they try to escape from, a friend told me that his own understanding of the condition his daughter suffered from came when it was pointed out that he suffers from claustrophobia . . . He knows claustrophobia is a nonsense, that the walls aren't really closing in, but in a tight spot he still feels an overwhelming panic anyway. It was pointed out that his daughter feels the same way about food, and it helped him empathise, rather than rage.

And then, somewhere early on in this journey to health, I came across the killer quote, from the great 18th-century English writer Samuel Johnson, 'Abstinence is as easy to me, as temperance would be difficult . . .'

BINGO!

That is exactly my position. And exactly the experience of so many of us.

Relying on your willpower to pull back every meal is hopeless. Sooner or later – by which I mean two days, max, Boomka – you will fall back into your old ways. Rather, you need to work out what is doing the damage, and then wipe it out entirely, exactly the way you – hopefully – wiped out tobacco and no longer miss it.

And I'll bet it will be yours if you just give it a chance . . .

But a brief pause here, as I suspect there needs to be space for many worthy and sincere experts tut-tutting, saying that a *much* better solution than going after unattainable abstinence is to *embrace moderation* in all things.

Hey, thanks, Scoop! Look, you make the coffee, and I'll hold the front page!

Of course they are dead right. But might I humbly and respectfully suggest that those experts *get* moderation, like you and I never will! And as it happens I am an expert on the inner psychology of big bastards who need to find a new approach to their inner conviction that **evermore food and grog = ever better**.

Have a look around at the local shopping mall. Or in your local mirror. How is all that moderated moderate moderation – a little bit of this and a little bit of that, and no I really shouldn't – going?

Not well? Interesting.

See, if you can master moderation, of *course* it is a ten times better and more sensible option than anything else! But it is beyond me, and I am guessing, Boomka, if your body weight got so far above what it should have been, and you have got through this book to this point, it has probably been beyond you, too?

The only way I got up to 152 Kegs – and you got, let's face it, to three-quarters of the weight of a heffalump, keep the change, love – was because even though I appreciated intellectually the virtues of easing back on everything, emotionally, spiritually and even philosophically, the truth is that, practically, that approach is as difficult to master as Chinese calculus.

So while I could go two days, three days and on a good week seven, being sensible, sooner or later – and usually sooner rather than later – I would go back to the old ways, praise the Lord and pass the party pies.

Who ate all the pies? You fat bastard, you fat bastard, you ate all the pies!

Actually, I did.

Hence the solution . . .

Instead of taking an excessive approach to eating and drinking, I just needed to change channels and apply that same tendency to an excessive passion for healthy rather than unhealthy things.

What about you at least try it, too? Turn your all or nothing approach from a weakness to a strength. So far, you've been taking the all approach with hot dogs and Kit Kats and beer, but see how you go with the nothing approach? It stands to reason that if you can give wolfing down a three-course meal and a bottle of wine everything you've got, then you've got the aptitude to do the exact opposite?

It's sort of like the horseshoe theory of politics, whereby those on the extreme left and extreme right often have an extraordinary commonality. I am the same man, gone from one side of the horseshoe diet to the other, with very little trouble – the difference being I am 45 kilos lighter. And herein, Boomka, is what I hope is the ever diminishing guts of this book.

For you and me, losing weight is *not* about pavlovas and Pinot Noirs and going easy on both – it's about parameters and principles, and putting them in place as part of our lives, so that by observing them, our weight sorts itself out, without us even having to think about it in detail at all.

It is understanding that the wankers – those who lectured us for years, that all diets are hopeless, because once you go back to your normal ways the weight goes straight back on, were . . . *what's that word again?* . . . RIGHT.

So let's go back to parameters.

Instead of all the tedious carry-on of working out how many kilojoules/calories in each meal, why not go with the big picture? Why not focus on knocking out whole food and drink groups, altogether?

Here is how it worked for me.

Start at go, with 152 kilos.

Knock out takeaway food, lose 12 kilos = 140 kilos.

Knock out sugar, lose the hunger, and eat sensibly, lose 12 kilos = 128 kilos.

Knock out grog, lose another ten kilos = 118 kilos.

Start going to the gym and jogging a bit obsessively, lose another six kilos = 112 kilos.

And we are *done*!

The virtues of this approach are exactly those delineated by Samuel Johnson, so I'll say it again.

'Abstinence is as easy to me, as temperance would be intolerable . . .'

Without sounding like a mad monk – I hope – I have found my rectitude liberating. Now that I have made the leap to abstinence, I need put no further time or any energy into every meal to work out what I should or shouldn't be eating or drinking. That job is done.

I already know: I avoid golden arches, I resist sugary stuff, I abstain entirely from alcohol, I get my arse moving. Case closed! Weight gone!

How *easy* is that?

Too easy, Campese.

I only wish I had sorted the whole thing out yonks ago.

Which brings us back to you. When do you think is the right time to start?

How bout . . . now?

If not you, who?

If not now, when?

The alternative, and you know it, is to go on with the bullshit diets and false-starts you have been on for the last few decades, and just getting ever bigger.

And that is no alternative at all.

So try this way instead?

Read on, mate.

TEN

Get moving!

'No matter how slow you go, you're still lapping everyone on the couch . . .'
Anon
(Love it!)

'A half-hour workout is only four per cent of your day.'
The trainers' aphorism

The other part of Gillespie's thesis where my approach has differed concerns what he wrote about physical activity:

'Don't exercise if your dominant purpose is to lose weight: let a lack of fructose do that instead. If you want to go for a walk or kick a ball, then go right ahead. If you don't feel like it, then don't do it.'

His broad point is that as 80 per cent of your weight is determined by your diet and only 20 per cent by what kind of exercise you do, the most important thing is to sort out your diet first and foremost.

Totally correct. And I might add that that rule is a neat reversal of the more famed 80/20 rule which says that, in life, 80 per cent of your happiness will come from just 20 per cent of your activities.

But again, my view is that just as the virtues of Gillespie's whole approach is that it steers our diet back towards what our natural intake is meant to be – and we feel better because of it – I would make the same claim about exercise. At various times in my life, I have suffered from a condition whereby the ramrod in my spine somehow gets magnetised . . . and exerts this extraordinarily powerful force whereby I am inexorably drawn to any couch within 50 metres.

I am going about my business, and then suddenly it has dragged me in, and I am pinned to the bloody thing! Can't move. The worst of it, of course, is that just as slugs breed more slugs, so does sluggishness breed more sluggishness, and it always takes an effort of will for me to get up off the couch and get moving again. But then, when I do, and get into regular exercise, just like learning to hate the taste of Coke, I come to hate sluggishness and want to get moving again.

So let's get to the exercise part.

My wise mate Dave the Dentist pointed out a couple of things to me about three years ago. 'Look at Kenny,' he said, 'he should be your model.'

Kenny is another tall mate of ours, in his late 60s, who, when we play touch football, runs like a giraffe bitten by a swarm of bees, leaving men up to 30 years his junior in his wake – and those men include me. He doesn't have an ounce of fat on him, and if I had to put the sheep station on one bloke I know living to 100 and having an active and engaged life all the way there, it would be Kenny.

The second thing Dave said was equally pertinent. 'All of us in our 40s, 50s and 60s,' he said, 'have a very clear choice. Move or die.'

His point was that nature's revenge on the truly sedentary who live lives that our bodies were simply not designed for – sitting around, doing three-fifths of fuck-all most days, and *four*-fifths of fuck-all on Sundays – is to make all the muscles we don't use wither and die. Sometimes, of course, it's the heart muscle. Other times it's the basic muscles that guide our movement.

You may remember the joys of team sport way back when? The time you kicked the winning goal, scored the half-century when your grandpa was watching, came second in the cross-country, or the day you ran the blind and scored in the corner right by the spot where your parents and grandma were standing?

My own game of choice was rugby, and one of my favourite quotes about the game goes like this (with thanks to Gerard Piper of Manly, who wrote this in the *SMH* Letters to the Editor, 1 July 1995): 'For boys it is the game for the sunshine of their lives, when the world is full and round and there is health and wonder in the air; a game of the mind as well as the body, and a test and source of character. Rugby football inspires all those qualities of skill and courage, magnanimity, co-operation and unselfishness that give the game its universal appeal to men of free spirit.'

I'm sure all sports have equally passionate quotes about the joys of their own code, but I love that quote for how well it encapsulates the exuberance of sporting youth, when the sun shone, and you could run all day with your mates.

My question to you is: do those really have to be bygone days? Why not get back involved in team sports now? Three of the great joys of my life in my 50s are playing basketball on Wednesday nights – we are not very skilled, but make every foul count – touch football with mates on three weekday mornings from 6.30 to 7.30, and tennis on the weekends. I am not particularly good at any of them, but oh, the joy, the fun, the mates, the time we beat the Legends with the three-pointer from Denis in the semis, with just two seconds left on the clock! And, quite seriously, while wild horses couldn't get me out of the house at 10.20 on a wet Wednesday night to get some exercise, I not only answer the call of the Lizards, I bloody well *make* the call: 'Come on, you bastards, we NEED you. We've got the Westsydaz tonight. We must beat them!'

As for touch football, of its many virtues it is not just playing with mates, it is making new ones as blokes from the whole area come and play.

Look around you, wherever you live. Those kinds of games will likely be taking place in some fashion, somewhere near to you.

Why not give it a go? I am particularly proud of the touch football game we play. Our oldest player is about 79, 'Old Pauly', and sometimes we have the ten-year-old son of one of the players, 'young Jackson', marking him. One of our players, when he was living in Australia, was Robbie Deans, the All Black fullback, who later became Wallaby coach. (I had been bitterly critical of his initial appointment to the Australian coaching role, until it was pointed out to me that it was actually just very nice to see a Kiwi living happily in Australia . . . with a job.) Another player was Joe Hockey, Federal Treasurer, frequently marked by one of Australia's long-term unemployed.

All up, a wonderfully Australian scene.

Beyond the virtues of raising a sweat, we are part of a very tight sporting community who, one way or another, look after each other. We attend weddings, parties, funerals, give each other advice on dealing with everything from teenagers to out-laws, and occasionally even steer work each other's way. Our wives know each other, and I can never walk down the main street near where we live without running into one or two of them and having a laugh. I tell you what, beyond everything that game does for our physical health, its effect on our mental health is immeasurable. When, sometimes, one or other of us might be going through a bad patch, Dave the Dentist is usually the first aware of it and does what he can to gently let those of us who need to know what is going on, so we can do what we can for them, or them for us.

I ain't turning this into an agony aunt column, but do you have that in your life? I believe it is important.

Even as we speak, just under half of all Australians between the ages of 16 and 85 have, at some point in their lifetimes, experienced a mental disorder, suffering everything from extreme anxiety to severe depression[1] – and it is utterly tragic. And while medication undeniably helps deal with some of it, one thing we know for sure is that regular exercise has an enormous impact on your mental state. I would maintain that exercise with mates, in a manner that *connects* you to your community, is the best tonic of all.

And, yes, I know you might be too busy for such malarkey . . . but are you really? For an Australian male, casual community sport can be the closest thing you are going to get to group therapy. Women, it seems to me, commendably talk to each other about personal things all the time, but men all too frequently don't. But we do play sport and get that spirit of camaraderie that comes along with it. Team-mates become mates very quickly. When you're away from work, away from family, away from your routine, you become for that hour a group of blokes playing sport just like you used to when you were a lad. Not particularly well, but it is fun . . . actual fun with exercise attached. Make the effort, it's worth it.

Another mate is one of Australia's most in demand and busiest barristers, who charges a fortune for every six minutes of consultation, so when he puts in an hour, three mornings a week, going cycling with mates, it directly comes off his billable hours and by that reckoning costs him thousands of dollars.

But his point to me is a beauty: 'An hour on the bike with my group is not an hour lost, it's an hour gained.' (I suspect President Barack Obama, also known to be busy, but still able to work in a 40-minute workout of some sort every day, justifies it on the same grounds.)

My mate means that if he lived his life by the reckoning that he would be losing money if he didn't always rip into the work that was there to do, he would never do anything else *but* work – and plenty of blokes do indeed fall into that trap. But by spending that time three mornings a week doing something he loves to do, and having coffee with his fellow cyclists afterwards, it clears his head, freshens him up, and makes him more productive in the long haul anyway.

A small parenthesis here. The one thing that does worry me about the cyclists is what they wear. When *I* go to play touch, I first engage in the traditional Australian male pastime of searching the bottom of the laundry basket and sorting through the crap in the back of my car, until I find what I am looking for: my scungy old footie shorts, my odd socks and my cleanest dirty T-shirt, usually one of many with food stains. And I play with and against blokes wearing much the same. But what the hell is it with the show-pony cyclists? Why, when we are dressed in scunge and grunge, just like our fathers taught us, and their fathers taught them, do each and every one of you look like you're trying out for the Tour de France fashion show? Every weekend! You set it all off with designer dark glasses and designer shoes – and I have the distinct impression that your entire outfits can be found in the one drawer at home, all neatly pressed and freshly washed, probably by a man-servant called Julio. And then you sit around in cafes for hours afterwards, looking like billboards for everything un-Australian. What is it with you people? But I digress. The main thing, I guess, is that at least you are out there, moving your bodies. Close parenthesis.

There is a difference between living and existing. Live a little, play some sport and make yourself live longer. I know you are not as good or as young as you once were, but neither is anyone else. Think on it. Actually, don't think on it, *do it*.

And look, if none of the above commends itself to you as an activity, at least get a pedometer which you can strap onto your belt to measure how many steps you take in a day. I first put one on via some promotion tagged to the great Australian runner Herb Elliott, when I was doing breakfast radio back in 2007 – a time when touch football in the mornings was an impossibility. The idea was 8000 steps a day for basic fitness and 10,000 steps to lose weight. The first day I did . . . 2000 steps! It was a wake-up call. Bit by bit, I managed to increase that to get it up to at least 8000 doing such things as walking to the shops instead of taking two tonnes of sleek machinery; walking the dog; walking back from basketball. Something, anything, but it helped change the way I lived and I was healthier. (Though still very heavy, as I had not yet got on to eliminating sugar.)

Still, one other thing while I have your attention on this. If you actually are losing weight and exercising more, you will, likely, be thrilled and you deserve to be. You might even start to idly wonder where you are on the 'BMI Index', if you've heard of that.

Your BMI is your Body Mass Index, and instead of being the ultra-modern bit of nonsense I thought it was, it goes back to 1835 when a Belgian bloke invented it – I believe his name was Marcel Index – and it is a way of measuring just where everyone fits on the slim-to-overweight scale. The formula relies on taking your weight in kilograms and dividing it by the square of your height in metres to come up with a number that fits on that scale. These days you get it by putting 'BMI index' into Google, and punching your own numbers into one of the many sites that come up and it's . . .

Depressing, yes?

Look, for me it was a double blow. First, while I thought 152 kilograms for 2.01 metres – 2.04 when I am in my high heels on a Saturday night – might get me to the borderline of obese, it was much worse than that. For, in fact, at a BMI of 37.62, I was so firmly in the postcode of obese, I was camped right next to its GPO, squeezed in between a Maccas and a KFC. A healthy BMI, they say, is between 18.5 and 24.9.

The second blow was that only after dropping 30 and a bit kilos did I finally move from the obese range into the overweight range. And that was dispiriting.

Now, down to 108 kilograms, I am still in the marginally overweight range but only just, and am encouraged to keep going.

Look, one thing you can console yourself with is that it doesn't actually measure lean muscle, so at the height of his powers when Arnold Schwarzenegger weighed 106.5 kilos and was 187.8 centimetres, it gave him a BMI of 30.5. This, according to the BMI Index, put him in the 'high health risk range' and classified him as 'obese'. Will Skelton of the Wallabies weighs in at 140 kilograms and is 203 centimetres tall. That gives him a BMI of 34.0, which would put him well into the high health risk range and close to very obese! Sam Thaiday of the Broncos, Queensland and Australia team, is one of the hardest, toughest footballers in Australia, but at 181 centimetres and weighing 112 kilograms, his BMI is 34.2 and he, too, is letting the side down as an obese man. So, mate, at least you and I have been in good company over the years!

Was Arnold Schwarzenegger depressed, incidentally, because he was technically obese? No. He kept his chin up, his standards down and kept making bad movies and impregnating the hired help. Okay, that's not the best example, but instead of depressing you, perhaps the BMI can inspire you?

In fact, it is a nice, solid, stubborn figure that gives you a good target to try to get down to. The BMI does not care that you think you look better, or that your jeans have a bit of give, or that you skipped dessert all last week. It is a cold, hard bastard of a drill sergeant that you can't argue with. If you are currently playing football for your country or co-starring in action movies you can argue with it, other-wise accept it and change.

I have come to the reluctant conclusion that we only think the target weight for men our height reads too low because our version of what is and isn't correct weight at Flemington – surrounded as we are by obesity (*sniff*) – is way too high. I reckon we must keep going anyway.

Whatever else, it is a great way of measuring flab when you apply it to an entire population.

On the BMI Index in 1995, 56 out of every 100 Australians were overweight or obese. In 2011, it had climbed to 63 out of every 100.[2] That's 11.2 million of us! We are heading to an extraordinary two-thirds of us being overweight within just a handful of years – and men are already there. A staggering 70.8 per cent of us are overweight right now, and the figure is climbing.

My man, this is an epidemic.

And we have to do our bit to stop it.

And if BMI doesn't totally work for you, try this as another measure: your waist–hip. Measure the number of centimetres of your waist at your belly button, and divide it by the number of centimetres around your bottom at its biggest. How did you go? A broad guide is, if you are fit and strong, it should be about 0.90. In my case, my waist is now 102 centimetres, my hips 106 centimetres, delivering a ratio of .96. I am getting there.

It is possible, just possible, that taking up exercise again will be easier than you think, for the very fact that normal size people actually want to move.

For me, once the weight started to drop, the old – by which I mean *young* – me, started to return. Without hauling 44 kilos of lard through the day and night, all day and night, every day and night, I felt completely different.

I realised that old, fat, slow feeling I had been getting in recent years was nothing of the sort. I wasn't old and fat and slow, I was merely fat and slow! And both of those conditions are rectifiable . . .

There had been times, true, in recent decades when the urge to go for a run or the like had suddenly possessed me, but on such occasions I was very strict – I would lie down on the couch and wait until the feeling had completely passed.

Now, I actually feel like going for a run for the sheer *fun* of it! And so I do. And then I go again. And again and again. Admittedly the old habits kicked in. I, of course, register my times for each run, and on successive runs I try to beat that time. I am, in case you haven't picked it up, competitive by nature. And who better to compete against than myself? And what better cause with which to harness that competitiveness than pursuing my own health?

It has even got to the point of going to the gym – despite me having sneered unpleasantly at the whole notion of gym junkies for most of the last 30 years.

(What is *wrong* with those people? Do they really have NOTHING better to do with their time? At least real junkies don't sweat all over their equipment. Urghh.)

It started with one of my mates from touch football and tennis, Gerard, insisting I go just once with him, where a young trainer by the name of Jess Cross would put us through our paces. My response to Gerard – as a real man – was, no, not interested. But he more or less wouldn't take, 'Get out of my face, bro'!' for an answer.

His key selling point?

'It's only 30 minutes.'

I reluctantly acquiesced. Sure enough, it was every bit as dull as I had feared. I lifted the free weights as Jess directed me, pushed and pulled on the machines, and did the various contortions – even as she noted down just what my limits were. All I cared about was getting out of there in 30 minutes, and lifting a bit more than Gerard, just on principle.

I hated . . . every . . . second . . . of it.

But, look, I did lift more than him. And I did go 15 metres further than him on the rowing machine in the allotted 60 seconds, not that I was counting – much.

And then, hold-the-phone, the strangest thing . . . For the rest of the day, my body sort of pleasantly *tingled*. In parts, I hurt, but I was aware that I had used muscles I hadn't used for 20 years and it just felt right. It played exactly into Dave the Dentist's 'move or die' line.

So when Jess called the next week, I reluctantly agreed to go back for another session – where I was a bit chuffed to have beaten all of the limits of the previous week, and a little interested if I could do it again next session – and I was soon hooked. The stronger I got, the more the 30 minutes whizzed by in nothing flat, and I soon mixed it up with hour-long sessions.

The most stunning thing of all?

After a few months I was demonstrably . . . wait for it . . . *growing* muscle. Instead of merely slowing the rate of decay as I had imagined gym work would be about at my age, I am, at the age of 55, actually getting *stronger*.

Who knew that was possible?

I did not.

At the time of writing – August 2016 – I have been doing it for seven months, and even in that space of time the number of kilograms that I can bench-press and dead-lift has more than doubled.

What is the point, you ask, when never in my ordinary life will I need to lift 85 kilograms off my chest, or lift a weight of 125 kilograms up to my knees? That is a legitimate question. And the answer is equally legit: I feel stronger. And everything else I do works better. In late June, two extra-ordinary things happened in the space of a couple of days: instead of my legs just being an amorphous mass of thunder thighs and lumpy calves as I was used to, they actually started to show muscly *shape*! Two days later, getting out of the shower, I spied, not quite my abs ... but very defi-nitely the shape of *an* ab beneath the flab! Two weeks later, a *second* ab showed up, as more flab diminished! No, I don't yet have a six-pack, and am not in it for that. (No, really.) But the satisfaction has been enormous. Plus there's that sense of strength.

Stunned as I was at seeing leg muscles and two abs, I resolved to work even harder, fastening my obsessive streak now ever more on working hard in the gym.

And it wasn't just for strength or the body beautiful alone.

For there is one other thing on this, if you are still with me.

Even in the Wallabies, I always thought the whole stretching thing was a wank. It might be all right for the likes of Carl Lewis, and I'd take his word for it that it might have shaved a few hundredths of a second off his time for the 100 metres – but that bloke was so finely tuned, so refined, it was said he would wear make-up when competing to look better for the camera.

Good luck to him. But for us footballers in the forwards? Please. We were tractors, not Maseratis, and that kind of fine-tuning was a bit beside the point.

Sure, I went along with it – when Alan Jones or Bob Dwyer were watching – and stretched my hammies the best I could, but never had my heart in it.

But now, friends, at long last, I get it!

Part of my same gym routine includes vigorous stretching and my whole body has now become ever more flexible. Beyond feeling stronger, I also feel somehow younger. I had forgotten that feeling of being able to move my body every which way, for long periods of time, and now I remember again. (And the make-up? *Love it!*)

If only I knew it back then. Somehow, the virtues of stretching were never properly explained to me. That's my excuse, anyway.

So let me explain it the way I now understand it. Each of our limbs has an arc of movement, with the limits of that arc determined by how far the muscles that move those limbs can stretch. The reason we are sore after physical effort is because we stretch those muscles to their natural limit and a little more, hence the hurt. But by stretching them beforehand, two things happen. The arc of movement gets greater, meaning we move more easily and we hurt less afterwards, meaning we can more quickly resume strong physical activity without hobbling around.

Oh, sure, it seems obvious to you. Doesn't every bastard know that?

No, actually, some of us didn't.

The point is, by taking stretching seriously for the first time in my sporting life, I have got so much more movement back it is frightening – at least it frightens the blokes on the other side of the net – *and* I am not sore the next day.

Yes, just like when I was young.

Weird. Why wasn't I told this? To be fair, I may have been told this but was probably absent at the tuckshop at the time. You will be amazed at how right fit people are if you actually try what they have been suggesting all along. It's almost like they knew what they were talking about.

Weird!

To finish this rant, I offer an analogy from Dr Rosemary Stanton. She notes that if a farmer leaves chooks and pigs and cattle to wander and eat at will, they won't get fat. But if you want to fatten those animals for market, then you have to put them in a confined space so that their appetite control goes haywire and they just eat and eat. Our modern lifestyle is like a big cage where we spend most of our lives sitting – usually near food.

Do you get it, Boomka?

Put down the donut, get out and wander the paddocks, jump over the fences, circle the trees, or you and the other pudgy porkers in the office will be buying the bloody farm a lot sooner than you should.

ELEVEN

Cooking up a storm

'Let food be thy medicine . . .'
Hippocrates

'Good food is very often, even most often, simple food.'[1]
from Kitchen Confidential: Adventures in the Culinary Underbelly by Anthony Bourdain

'I always think if you have to cook once, it should feed you twice. If you're going to make a big chicken and vegetable soup for lunch on Monday, you stick it in the refrigerator and it's also for Wednesday's dinner . . .'
Curtis Stone, Australian chef

Yes, I know it's borderline, but when I lived in France for four years in the 1980s – living in the village of Donzenac, while playing rugby for the nearby town of Brive – a Gypsy friend of mine always delighted in telling me his recipe for *la soupe des Gitans*, 'Gypsy soup'.

'*Tout d'abord*,' he would say, '*voler un poulet*.'

First of all, steal a chicken.

Boom-boom.

For you and me, mate, would I be right in saying that for the better part of our lives our major contribution to getting dinner on the table is either saying to our mothers, wives or girlfriends, 'What's for dinner?' and then sometimes having a grizzle when it is not to our liking?

I, at least, am guilty as charged. And for a lot of us who got huge, at least one part of the problem was leaving home without the first clue as to how to cook for ourselves like a grown-up, meaning that a constant recourse was takeaway, am I right?

That, too, was me.

Three things, however, helped me heaps on this journey to health.

The first, oddly enough, was that stint in France, home of the finest cuisine on earth. And that fine cuisine included, to my amazement, salad!

Ah yes, as a down-home Australian lad, I thought I knew all there was to know about salad. Growing up on the farm, salad was the few stray, sad little leaves Mum sometimes put beside the meat and three vegies. And when we inevitably didn't eat it, my frugal mother would gather them in, put them in the fridge until the next lunch or dinner. Mum was so big on leftovers it was never remarked upon in our house and, as the old gag goes, there was some quiet conjecture as to what the original meal must have been, and from what decade it might have dated?

Mum's commitment to never throwing food out – displaying the extreme frugality that Grandpa had taught her – was so strong that very occasionally it got to the point that not even Dad could stand it.

I mean, he could eat week-old mashed potato and beans with the best of them, he didn't mind soup or stew that had already been re-warmed four or five times, but . . .

But on one famous family occasion, when Mum thought the only way out from throwing away a week-old salad was to boil it and serve it as one would cabbage, Dad finally had enough. 'I'm sorry, dear,' he said, pushing the plate away from him, 'but I *cannot* eat this.'

Entirely unfazed, Mum simply scraped the mess from Dad's plate onto her own, and stoically worked her way through the whole thing.

Let's face it, the stray bit of lettuce was the kind of 'salad' I, and many Australians of our generation, grew up with.

But when I went to live in France, it was . . . different. For starters, the salad was always fresh. And mixed with other things like slices of *fromage* and *tomate* and this fabulous ham, *jambon de Bayonne*.

And – for this was the most important thing of all – the whole salad was lightly covered in this extraordinarily delicious thing called *vinaigrette*. My favourite was a light mix of olive oil, balsamic vinegar, garlic and mustard.

A whole new world opened up. For the French on a good day, salad is not the thing on the side, it is the whole freaking meal, and it is *fabulous*. And there was absolutely nothing of the notion that only namby-pamby ninnies ate salad. My friend, and the flanker of our team, Christian Dalla-Riva – one of the hardest, toughest bastards I've ever met, and I've met and fought with a few – pretty much *only* ate salad through the summer months. And, of course, he had not an ounce of fat on him, seemingly to be made mostly of bone, gristle, knees and elbows.

Whatever else, it made me understand just how delicious salad could be and killed off the very last of my absurdly provincial notion that while Real Men Don't Eat Quiche, they never, *ever*, eat salad. Given that Christian was so tough – he once took on damn nigh the entire pack of the tearaway Toulon team on his own – and he was great in the kitchen, it also helped me through the tragic nonsense that real men don't cook.

And since learning about the damage done by sugar, I've had cause to look at my French experience with fresh eyes.

You may recall there was a fantastically popular book a few years ago called *French Women Don't Get Fat*. I've been thinking about that book lately. In all of my time in that village, in all my many trips all over France – and I have been back at least once a year ever since – you just don't see obese women, and very few obese men. And yet, in *La Republique Francaise,* we ate and drank like royalty! The cuisine was superb, and taking time to sit at the table and enjoy the meal was sacrosanct. But . . . what we were all eating was whole food. Freshly prepared, most often freshly grown, there was of course no fast food culture in my village, no obsession with throwing vast quantities of soft drink down your gullet when a glass of superb Bordeaux is cheaply available and hits the spot just as it has for their forebears for centuries.

Incidentally, while back in Donzenac in July of 2016, I mentioned to my friend Mousse, who commented on my newly svelte form, that I had entirely stopped drinking wine since discovering that one bottle of wine is equivalent to eating a Big Mac.

He looked at me, aghast.

'*Mais,*' he spluttered, '*qui se tape une bouteille entière de pinard d'un coup?*' But, who would knock back a whole bottle of wine in one go?'

What sort of gauche dickhead would *ever* do that?

I shifted uncomfortably.

Another French friend, Presia, who has lived in Australia for the last 25 years, was shocked when coming here to see the quantities of food we habitually pile on our plate.

Eating and drinking with *care* – neither gulping nor guzzling – is simply in their blood and because they're not sluicing sugar syrup through their system every day, their bodies look after the rest, naturally. They dinkum *do* stop when they've had an elegant sufficiency.

For that matter, I thought about my time living in Italy for a year, also playing rugby, in the town of Rovigo, just south of Venice. In that town, then and now, obesity is just about unknown. What do they eat? Pasta. What does pasta consist of? The staple ingredient is glucose.

With no fructose as part of that staple, their bodies self-regulate.

Now, it is true, once I returned to Australia I didn't particularly take up eating salad, or cooking heaps, but it set me up for what happened just over 20 years later, when I was embarking on getting healthy again.

A notably slim friend, Ali, told me I needed to have a 'go-to meal', something I could whip up in no time at all that was healthy for me. And she even gave me the perfect example, in little words that even I could understand.

Grab a whole bunch of rocket, or mixed leaf salad. Sprinkle lightly with balsamic vinegar. (David Gillespie, however, insists that as balsamic vinegar has a 15 per cent sugar content – again I say, *who knew?* – 'better to go with olive oil and lemon juice, with a bit of salt and pepper if you insist'.) Then get some pine nuts and lightly roast them, and finally get some thinly sliced pieces of halloumi cheese that you sear in a fry pan or on a sandwich maker. Mix the whole lot together and who is your uncle?

Bob!

It tastes delicious, has no more than a *soupçon* of sugar and you can make it in five minutes, tops. If you make enough for your wife and kids – I know, I know, the idea of *you* cooking for the family might be blowing your mind right now, but anyway – they can have it too, and I promise you, they will love it!

And you really do need to have a go-to meal, just like that. A couple of the recipes below might help, with the virtue that you can make a heap of them, put the remains in the fridge and they will taste every bit as good – and be every bit as healthy – when you warm them up throughout the week.

The other thing that changed for me was receiving instructions from my wife and daughter that during said daughter's HSC, dinner would henceforth be on the table at 7 pm sharp, so she could build her study schedule around it, and that *I* was the cook. (Which was fair enough as my missus does breakfast television, and it was high time I dipped my oar in and began to pull my weight.) The added complication was that as my daughter is a vegetarian, it was a fairly obvious step for me to make meat-free meals that Lisa and I could enjoy, too, and the consequence was that my meat intake was hugely reduced.

And blow me down if the weight didn't fall off once more!

Look, I don't want to get into the whole vegetarian/ meat-eating debate, because as you will have noted in the discussion above, you can eat healthily with or without meat. But I will say this: since going through that whole HSC period a significant light went on in my head: I simply didn't need the huge slabs of meat I was eating every day. A vegetarian meal was every bit as good, if you know what you're doing. Now, as it happened, I didn't, but my vegetarian son, Jake, did, and he helped me get my head around it, just as he helped with this book.

Meantime the Brownie points of cooking for your family – just like a grown-up – are *not* to be underestimated.

Before you dismiss it, just give it a shot. And remember, I know at least enough about cooking to have once appeared on *Celebrity MasterChef* with the likes of Michelle Bridges, and was *very* unlucky to be pipped at the post by her! But don't get me started . . .

Now, believe me, this next recipe is cheap as chips (but much less fattening), and as healthy as jogging. It will put some lead in your pencil to boot, which, I repeat, you are going to need now that you are the hero of the house once more. Best of all, you can have bowl after bowl and it's going to put bugger-all pressure on your waistline. It's not going to raise cholesterol, it's free of butters and oils and – if you care – the fat content is non-existent! It has a bit of salt, but it's a negligible amount. And, of course, no sugar!

You might be asking, 'Without any of that, how can it taste good?' The trick is the spices. Paprika, chilli and garlic will do you no harm but give you a full, rich flavour with enough kick that you'll savour every mouthful.

(This, by the by, is what my son Jake has taught me lies at the heart of a lot of healthy cooking. You take both sugar *and* fat content away from a meal, and then save it from blandness through the spices. Think of it as . . . *sophisticated* cooking.)

Good luck . . .

Bean and Veggie Soup

Tools:

A big pot

A good knife and chopping board

A colander/strainer/bucket full of holes

The right attitude (*Come on*, you bastard. Try it, just once. And trust me. Remember – I was on *Celebrity MasterChef!*)

Ingredients:

800 grams frozen vegetables (You're looking for broccoli, carrots and cauliflower here, but whatever you can get in the frozen food section will cut it. Ignore my previous advice that bugger-all that comes in a packet is without sugar. This is a rare exception.)

2 × 420 gram tins of mixed beans (borlotti, kidney, cannellini, chickpea, whatever you've got)

6–7 cups of vegetable stock (If it looks like it needs more juice, throw a bit more on.)

420 gram tin of diced tomatoes

4 cloves of garlic (I love garlic, but adjust according to your own tastes.)

2 medium-sized potatoes (No need to skin them.)

1 onion (red, white, brown, who cares? Not me, and not you.)

400 grams fresh spinach. (Wash it if that stuff matters to you, but it's no big deal.)

Spices:

Pepper

Salt

Tabasco sauce
Paprika
Dried oregano

Optional:
Chilli flakes

Instructions:
1. Empty the whole bag of frozen vegetables right into the pot. No need to thaw them or chop them, just chuck them in directly from the freezer.
2. Put all the beans in a colander, rinse them with plenty of cold water to get rid of the thick juice and then throw them right into the pot as well.
3. Grab your onion, peel and dice it. Doesn't need to be perfect, but you don't want big pieces. Throw it in the pot.
4. Grab your potatoes and dice them. You want pieces smaller than the size of the end of your little finger. Throw it all in the pot.
5. Chop up your garlic and throw it in the pot. The smaller the pieces the better, but no stress either way.
6. You should now be looking at a pot full of raw vegetables and beans. It might not look like much, but it's about to.
7. Pour in all six cups of vegetable stock.
8. Throw in a pinch of salt, a pinch of pepper, a pinch of oregano, a dash of Tabasco sauce and a heaped teaspoon of paprika.

9. Turn the heat on to high, and keep your eye on it. Stir occasionally. You want it to come to a boil but not stay there too long. Once you see bubbles and steam, turn down the heat until it's on a nice simmer. Throw in the tomatoes, give it a good stir and put the lid on.

10. You've got about 20 minutes now. That's the perfect amount of time to register as a member of the Australian Republic Movement. Just google us, go to the Membership link and tell them Pete sent ya.

11. Take the lid off and give it a taste test. What does it need? More flavour? Add more salt and maybe some cracked pepper. More kick? Throw in a bit of paprika and Tabasco. If you're happy with the flavour, move to the next step.

12. Throw in the spinach. It won't take long for it to wilt and blend with the rest of the soup, and once it has, you're ready to eat!

All Together Now:
Serve in a big bowl with toast or wholegrain bread on the side. Top each serve with a little grated parmesan, *et voila*!
Are you the hero of the house, and a BIG chance tonight?
One more then . . .

Bean Mix with Brown Rice and Fresh Salsa

More beans. I know. There's a reason I keep suggesting them. They're high in protein, fibre, iron and all the other healthy goodies you need to stay fit and healthy. (They also stop you needing to spend half an hour on the loo. And don't pretend you don't know what I'm talking about.)

This recipe also contains brown rice, and we should look at rice the same way we look at bread. The whiter it is, the less nutrient dense it is. By going with brown rice, we keep all the vitamins, iron and essential good stuff. I also prefer the nuttier flavour and texture that seems to keep me fuller for longer, but that's just me. The salsa is just fresh juicy tomato and cilantro (coriander, but you'll feel more like a ridgy-didge chef if you call it *cilantro*. Say it with me: sill-an-tro). And you can't have too many fresh veggies.

Tools:
A good knife and chopping board
A non-stick frying pan or small pot
Colander

Bean mix ingredients:
2 × 400 gram tins of kidney beans or mixed beans
1 brown onion
1 green/red/yellow capsicum
1 × 200 gram tin of diced tomatoes
2 cloves garlic
Dash of olive oil

Salsa ingredients:
1 clove of garlic
Handful of fresh cilantro
5 tomatoes
1 red onion
1 small lime

Rice ingredients:
1 cup of brown rice (roughly 400 grams)
2 cups of water
Pinch of salt

Spices:
Paprika
Ground cumin
Chilli flakes
Tabasco sauce
Pepper
Salt

Instructions:
1. Drizzle – *that is a great word we serious, kick-arse chefs use to mean 'pour'* – some olive oil in your frying pan.
2. Dice your brown onion and garlic. Fine small pieces are what we want. Into the pan they go.
3. Dice your capsicum. They don't have to be as small as the onion pieces, but not too big either. Into the pan!
4. Rinse and drain your beans in a colander.
5. Turn the heat on to medium and stir frequently. Stir in a dash of salt and a dash of pepper.
6. Once the onion and capsicum have started to brown a little and your kitchen starts to smell like you know what you're doing, throw in the mixed beans!
7. Continue to stir with the beans added, and throw in a teaspoon of paprika, cumin and half a teaspoon of chilli flakes. Keep on stirring periodically.

8. After five minutes, give it a test. Are the beans at a nice texture? If so, move straight to step 9. If not, give it a little more time. Likewise, if it's not hot enough or a tad bland, add salt, pepper or whatever else you feel is missing.

9. Throw in the diced tomato and give it enough time for the whole mixture to heat up, but not so long that the beans turn into mush.

10. Give it another taste test, and if you're happy, the bean mix is ready!

For the salsa:

1. Dice the tomatoes. This can be a bit difficult because of how watery they are, but a good chop will do.

2. Dice the red onion, as fine as you can.

3. Chop up the cilantro.

4. Slice the lime into quarters. Set aside for a second.

5. Dice the garlic.

6. Throw all of it into a bowl and give it a good stir. Don't be afraid to mash it up, just make sure it's thoroughly mixed in together. Squeeze the lime over the top of it and give it a last mix.

7. Your fresh salsa is complete!

Cooking your rice:

1. Throw your rice into a pot.

2. Cover the rice with water, add a pinch of salt.

3. Bring to a boil uncovered.

4. Once it's at a proper roiling boil, take it down to a simmer and put the lid on.

5. Leave it simmering for about 20 minutes, then turn off the heat completely.

6. Leave the rice to soak for another ten minutes, no heat applied and then it's ready!

All together now:

Now to make it into something that looks like a meal. You want your plate to be 50 per cent beans, 30 per cent brown rice and 20 per cent salsa. This is a bloody filling meal that will give you a heap of energy. Don't go crazy with seconds, though, because delicious as it is, it's a hearty meal.

Omelette/Scrambled Eggs with Cottage Cheese and Salmon

Omelettes don't really have a healthy reputation. That's because every amateur chef likes to throw everything they can think of/anything that is left in the fridge and about to go off, into a pan then toss two eggs on top of it, stir twice and call it an omelette. That's not an omelette, that is a mess. Now pay attention, 007, and learn the secret of a healthy omelette.

Tools:

Frying pan

Chopping board and knife

Bowl

A whisk (but a fork will do, as, seriously, this isn't *MasterChef*. Did I mention . . . ah, forget it.)

Ingredients:

3 eggs
A dash of milk
¼ capsicum
Little handful of red onion
Little bit of garlic
100 grams of salmon/smoked ocean trout
Spoonful of cottage cheese
Drizzle of olive oil

Instructions:

1. Crack your eggs and throw them in the bowl. Pierce the yolk with a fork, add a dash of milk, and whisk until it has a fairly uniform light yellow colour.
2. Dice your capsicum, throw it in.
3. Dice your red onion, throw it in.
4. Dice your garlic, throw it in. (Yeah, there's a pattern developing.)
5. Throw in your spoonful of cottage cheese and give the whole thing another whisk.
6. Dice your olive oil. Okay, that's a joke. *Drizzle* a little bit of olive oil in your frying pan and turn it to medium to high heat. Then throw the whole mixture in, trying to spread it from one side of the pan to the other.
7. Once it's evenly distributed over the frying pan, leave it and return to the chopping board.
8. Chop up your salmon/smoked trout and evenly distribute it over the top of the omelette. It's already cooked and heats up quickly, that's why we add it last.

9. Now for the only tricky part. Try to flip the omelette. In the somewhat likely event that it falls apart, don't stress. Just take whatever you were using to flip and break the whole thing apart. Keep smashing and separating it until it starts to look like scrambled eggs. Then guess what, you made scrambled eggs! Nobody will know the difference, least of all your stomach or taste buds.

All together now:

Not much more to say. Whack it all on a plate, maybe include a handful of English spinach leaves if you feel like some greens. (You can never have too much.) The best part is, this is a meal that will keep you trucking throughout the day. Now don't get me wrong, this is a hearty breakfast. If you're really trying to cut down your caloric intake, one change you can make is to separate the yolk from the eggs, and discard the yolk. (Am I serious? Yes. No yolk!) This is pretty easy: just try to crack closer to the tip and transfer the contents back and forth between the half shells without letting the yolk fall into your mix. This is what we call in the trade an Egg White Omelette.

One last thing. Once you've achieved your goal weight, I offer the following as an expert guide to how you should apportion a balanced meal. It comes from Dr John Berardi, who has a PhD in Precision Nutrition, on the subject of *Portioning the Perfect Meal*, from his book, *Create the Perfect Meal with This 5-step Guide*:

Portions for Male
Protein: 2 palms
Vegetables: 2 fists
Carb: 2 cupped hands
Fat: 2 thumbs
(Yes, you're right – a great rule of thumbs.)
And sugar in that? *Exactly.* No mention!

TWELVE

Ringing in the changes . . . unless you still don't get it?

'It's a terrible thing, I think, in life to wait until you're ready. I have this feeling now that actually no one is ever ready to do anything. There is almost no such thing as ready. There is only now. And you may as well do it now. Generally speaking, now is as good a time as any.'
Hugh Laurie, English actor

'People's ignorance really pisses me off. Stupidity is when you can't help it – ignorance is when you choose not to understand something.'
Sarah McLachlan, Canadian singer/songwriter

'Certainly, fat and sugar would be more to one's taste; in fact, those seem to me to be the great stand-by for one in this extraordinary continent; not that I mean to depreciate

*the farinaceous food, but the want of sugar and fat in all
substances obtainable here is so great that they become
almost valueless to us as articles of food, without the
addition of something else.'*
(Signed) W J Wills.
**The last words in the diary of William John Wills – of Burke
and Wills fame – just before he died of starvation, in June 1861**

Okay, so let's go through this.

The first and most crucial thing, mate, is to follow this
simple plan, bit by bit, to live a new, healthier life. We can
do this *togevva*, bro! You were decades on the path that took
you to this point, but if you get into it, you are about to be
amazed about how quickly you can turn this all around and
how forgiving – if you treat it nicely – your body can be.

Seriously, it is staggering. After *decades* of abuse, in
just a few concentrated months, you can undo much of the
damage. How is that possible? Because, this time, instead of
working against nature, sluicing crap through your system
that was never meant to be there, you will have the power
of nature at your back, the wind behind you, as your body
starts to transform itself back into the shape that nature
always intended.

So here's what to do now:

1. **Stop the sugar.**
   Stop the hunger. Be ruthless about what you put in
   your mouth. **Don't eat sweet.** Don't drink it, either. Move
   away from processed food to natural food. Get this into

your melon: if the food you are eating is processed, then four times out of five it has got sugar in it and, likely, *heaps* of sugar. And in that case there is three-fifths of bugger-all chance it will do anything but make you *more* hungry. Once you stop the sugar, it is an absolute revelation how the hunger fades. If you get nothing else from this book, get that. But what I have also realised is that you need to, effectively, listen to your body. That is, a lot of blokes find it nigh on impossible after yonks of tucking into three big meals a day – because that's what you do, right? – to push the plate back when there is still food on it. Nor do they get the concept of skipping the formal sit-down dinner and making do with something light, some fresh fruit or veggies or nuts after having had a big lunch. Dinner-time means *dinner*-time, and they are going to have DINNER, come hell or high water. But, particularly for older men with grown children – where meal-times are less part of the familial fabric – if you can get into the habit of munching on a couple of carrots instead of the whole enchilada, *skip the palaver and hold the pavlova*, the benefits are enormous.

2. Stop eating takeaway.

When I first got to grips with the damage takeaway was doing to me, the simple expedient of *not* putting my left blinker on every time I saw golden arches up ahead on the horizon stripped a good six kilos off me in as many months. What the hell was I thinking, so frequently dropping by for a mid-afternoon snack of large Coke,

Filet-o-Fish, Big Mac and large fries, and then being surprised I had put on so much weight? That 'meal' contains 1473 calories. Measure that against the fact that the average calories burned every day by an adult male are around 2200.

3. Get off the grog.

Think clearly, and stop being a piss-head. It is not just the damage it does in the calories it has, and everything else it does to your body, it is that it weakens your self-discipline in making good choices. Here endeth the sermon!

4. Take up some regular form of exercise.

Jog if you must (so long as you are not so heavy right now it's dangerous to do so without the okay from your doctor), otherwise find a regular physical activity with mates so that engaging in it gives you a reward for doing it, beyond your own virtue. *Move*, you bastard!

5. Measure that activity.

If you're running around in basketball or touch football or the like, wear a pedometer to see how many steps you do in the given time. Note it down. Give yourself something to push past next time. If swimming or jogging, note down your time over a given distance. This is particularly effective if you happen to be a competitive bastard, as when you're competing against yourself, you know your opponent is smart, tough and resilient, not to mention handsome, and you are going to have to make an extra effort to best him. Ultimately, you will be inspired as you see your stats improve.

6. Sleep properly!

For starters, people who wake up tired are likely to make poor choices. If you're tired, slow and grumpy, you're more inclined to want something immediately gratifying like a donut or, even worse, skip breakfast entirely, be ravenous by mid-morning, and blow the whole thing wide open. Whereas if you're well rested when you wake up, you're more inclined to have an apple and a piece of vegemite toast.

Why are we unusually hungry after a bad night's sleep, by the way? Because lack of sleep stuffs up your whole hormone system. You will recall I mentioned earlier in Chapter 5 about the hormones that control our hunger? Leptin gives you the full feeling, while ghrelin makes your tummy rumble, and makes you feel hungry. As discussed, sugar makes you resistant to the appetite suppressing hormone leptin, meaning you keep eating long after your body has had its fill. And lack of sleep does the same thing! Waking up after not enough sleep sees your leptin low and your ghrelin high. Added to that, the grumpiness that goes with lack of sleep makes us more inclined to grab something immediately gratifying to snap us out of it. Enter the Coco-Pops, *just like a milk-shake, only crunchy* AND twice the calories! Thereafter, throughout the day, much the same dynamic applies. With less sleep, complex decisions like, 'That slice of cake at the coffee shop looks really good but I'm trying to be conscious of what I eat so I'm going to avoid it and just have some wholemeal toast' are a lot harder than simple decisions like 'Cake? Me like cake. I eat cake.'

7. Weigh yourself, every morning.

Get one of those apps like *MyFitnessPal*, on your phone, to register the weight, to graph it, *every day*. And yes, yes, yes, I know that most dietitians say you shouldn't weigh yourself more than once a week, but they don't get our mentality quite the way we do. In my case I have always loved the line, *'I kept reading that smoking causes cancer, so I've stopped reading!'* And haven't you and I had a tendency over the years to be like that when it comes to checking our weight? Hasn't it so hurt us over the years every time we get on the scales, and see the awful truth, that we've steered away from such a gauche and vain practice ever since? Come on, you know it's true. And so we have to change that habit. NOTHING keeps you as honest on a Saturday night when the party pies are being passed around and the ice-cream handed out, as knowing you must face the tyranny of the scales of justice the very next day. And nothing is as wonderfully encouraging as seeing your numbers go down day by day, week by week, and seeing your graph starting to look like the main slope at Thredbo. (Which can be a bastard for a fat man, but a joy for your slimmer version.) It is energising! So get into it. Weigh yourself every morning – post ablutions, as if there is any other way, am I right, and register it. And don't skip days. If you break out on Maccas, if you give in and have the apple pie with ice-cream for dessert, face the pain the next day! I am telling you, it keeps you honest. (As tragic as it might sound, on a recent fortnight holiday in Europe, I took my home scales with me. Result? Instead of getting back two kilos heavier, as was usual, I made Correct Weight the first day back.)

8. **Change your daily habits and work out ways to avoid temptation.**

For example, former NSW Premier Bob Carr, always svelte, has a standing order every time a hotel room is booked in his name: *empty the mini-bar.* Brilliant. Personally, I've never understood how all those chippies and choccies always seem to know not just my name, but precisely the way to whisper it seductively, the moment I enter the room. Getting the hotel to banish them before I arrive, solves the problem.

9. **Slow your eating down so you can more properly judge when you are full.**

You are not in some sort of secret one-man eating competition. Seriously, *Oliver Twist* was just a book, nobody is going to grab your plate away. Do not be afraid to chew before you swallow. Always remember Tennessee Williams choked to death (yes, on the cap of a bottle of eye drops, but still the principle is the same). And the physiological reason is strong. Leptin can take as long as 15 minutes to kick in. The slower you are, the more chance you have to read your body's signals.

10. **Before heading out to a place where they're going to be serving *hors d'oeuvres*, party pies and so forth, *eat an apple*.**

    Make sure that your tummy is full before you get there, with good stuff, so you're less inclined to blow out on the bad stuff. An even better alternative is a handful of unsalted nuts, or better still, a carrot.

11. **Make sure you stay hydrated!**

    Short of drowning yourself, water is the ONLY thing that you cannot have too much of. And before every meal, and during it, drink at least a couple of glasses. Not only will it help with the feeling of fullness, but the entire process of digestion, and then moving the food through your body, is aided by it.

12. **Use smaller plates.**

    You'll put less food on your plate and you'll trick yourself into thinking that you're eating more. Seriously, the small plate thing works – and I know I'm repeating myself, but it's important. Our plates have been super-sized along with our stomachs. Change this. It's a simple mind game that actually works.

13. Eat mindfully.

Pay more attention to your food and less attention to your phone, the paper, the TV. If you can focus on what you eat, you'll be much more aware of what, and what amount, you're putting in your body. A fair guide for me has been that when, at the end of the day, I can remember everything I have eaten or drunk, it is a fair reckoning that I have eaten carefully, not wantonly.

14. Eat more veggies.

This does *not* mean more French fries. And you can ignore the fact, please, that in the US, tomato sauce is officially regarded as a vegetable for school lunches, and amounts are regulated! This means more good, wholesome vegetables. Carrots, broccoli, capsicum, corn, cauliflower, peas, it doesn't matter. Just get vegetables into you. Vegetables are packed to the brim with the vitamins and minerals that your body needs. Like I said, I'm no scientist or dietitian, so I can't tell you much about the vitamins and minerals, I just know they're good for you. What I do know, and what I can speak with authority on, is satiety. Vegetables have a very low caloric load. What they are is filling. Vegetables will fill you up like nothing else. You'll feel full as a goog, but you won't have actually eaten that much. Ergo, you will lose weight!

15. Don't drink sugary drinks.

I'm hoping that you've picked up on that by now, but just to reiterate . . . don't drink sugary drinks! Aside from the incredibly fattening nature of the sugar in those drinks, the fructose will suppress your ability to determine when you're full. And by the way, be wary of artificially sweetened drinks too. Yes, you're cutting your calories, but your tastebuds are still being left to crave sweetness. And you will reach for some sweet food to go along with your diet drink pretty fast to 'reward' your good behaviour. *Man up*, my man, and kick the whole damn thing.

16. Never, EVER go to the supermarket hungry.

This makes an enormous difference. Think about it. When you're hungry and surrounded by every possible food product on God's green earth, your willpower doesn't stand a chance! Doritos half price? Sure. Caramel Tim Tams on sale? We can make room. Cream cheese dips two for the price of one? That'll go well with the Doritos. If you're going to the supermarket with an empty stomach, it's just not a fair fight. Instead, go shopping after a decent meal and a big glass of water. You'll feel full, and instead of falling for the Cherry Ripes at the checkout, you'll realise you don't need any of that. This brings me to my follow-up point . . .

17. Go to the supermarket with a 'list'.

Instead of wandering around aimlessly and grabbing a frozen pizza, go to the supermarket with an itemised plan for what you actually need. Milk, eggs, wholegrain bread, garlic and two cans of beans? Get exactly that, pay for your produce, and head home. Remember:

you can't give in to the temptation of the Maltesers in the fridge at home if you never bought any in the first place.

18. If I can't talk you into giving the grog a rest, at least try to lower the calories!

Spirits have far fewer calories per standard drink than either wine or beer. Having said that, don't make the mistake of thinking rum & Coke is better than a glass of Sauvignon Blanc. The rum's not the problem, it's (you guessed it!) the Coke. Try spirits and sparkling water or club soda. If you can stomach it, have it on the rocks! This is just another little change that will have a big impact on your *not so little waistline*.

19. I've said it before and I'll say it again, you need to change your mentality.

Admittedly, this is a pretty big thing to do, and it may not happen overnight. But when you're struggling, when you really want to rip into a bucket of KFC, when you're wondering if maybe just a couple of chocolate bars would be all right, when you just NEED a can of Coke, remember this: *you're not on a diet. You're CHANGING your diet.* You're making a change that is going to inspire your kids, that's going to help you sleep better – not to mention more often with your wife or partner – a change that's going to help you move faster, that's going to help you think clearer. You're getting healthy, and it's admirable.

20. Remember, it's okay to feel a little hungry.

For the vast majority of human history, all the way from monkeys swinging from vine to vine, to cavemen, to pioneers, to struggling farmers, we have been just a tad hungry. It's the natural state. And if you're feeling a little hungry, what does it mean? It means your body is looking for food, and if you don't feed it, where will it look? It will look at itself. Yep, your very own body is a cannibal and you didn't even know it! Your body will look to your fat reserves and use them for energy. The sensation of hunger is the sensation of weight loss! Of course you don't have to be hungry all the time, but it is no bad thing when it does happen. Learn to embrace it.

THIRTEEN

The lines that stick

'You can't outrun a bad diet . . .'
Anon

'A man's health can be judged by which he takes two at a time – pills or stairs.'
Joan Welsh, Democratic Member of the US House of Representatives

'If man made it, don't eat it.'
Jack LaLanne, the self-described 'Godfather of modern fitness', who hosted the first fitness show on TV, starting in 1953 and continuing for 32 years. (And he's our kind of bloke. At the age of 54 – RAH! – he beat a 21-year-old Arnold Schwarzenegger in a push-up and chin-up contest at Venice Beach.)

Studying a few law subjects at Sydney Uni in the early 1980s, I guess I must have sat through – and sadly, for me, often slept through – 400–500 hours total of law lectures. And what did I retain of actual facts? About three-fifths of bugger-all. But I did grasp something far more important still, and that is a few legal principles. I learned, for example, that for a contract to be valid, there must be an *offer*, and that offer must receive *acceptance*. And finally for the contract to be valid, there must be *consideration* – the exchange of something, like money or goods or both, to confirm that a legal agreement has been reached.

It is the sort of dead simple principle that, once you get it in your melon, can guide you for the rest of your life in dozens of situations. Similarly, when I worked on building sites, I learned the Carpenter's Creed – *measure twice, cut once*. Grasp that, and you are halfway home to avoiding colossal stuff-ups. Savvy professional golfers have long noted, '*You drive for show, you putt for dough,*' and construct their training regimens accordingly. In my own world of the media for the last three decades, I have loved the line from the founder of Triple M, Rod Muir, '*If it ain't happening in the corridors, it don't go up the stick,*' the idea being that unless your team all genuinely like each other, you ultimately won't be able to fake a happy show going up the antenna of the radio or TV station that brings the punters in. Environmentalists, and that should be us all, say the mantra we must embrace is '*Think globally, act locally.*' In rugby, the firm rule was, '*Don't make Buck Shelford angry, or he'll rip you apart.*' (It didn't always work – even calm, he generally ripped us a new one, anyway.)

Now, I reckon getting into healthy eating and drinking and exercise is much the same for you and me. If we can just grasp a few solid principles to guide us, together with a few good lines that neatly encapsulate those principles, the rest will sort itself out. Because even if you embrace just a couple of these simple principles you will see progress. And once you start to see how far you can get by just tweaking your approach in those small ways, you may well get a bit addicted to it like I did – even *before* the Brownie points from your wife start rolling in, and you get to live out the most sacred principle of all for men our age, the aforementioned *'Happy wife, happy life!'*

Stay with it, and you're going to want more and more progress. You're going to want better results, you're going to demand more of yourself!

And because we have the attention span of a gnat, we need them in bite-size chunks that go down easy as an oyster, like, *'Nothing tastes as good as healthy feels.'*

Here are a few more:

- Growing up, the line against eating too much chocolate was this 'un: *'In your mouth for two seconds, your tummy for two hours and on your gut for two years.'* Or *'A moment on the lips, a lifetime on the hips.'* Got it? Brief pleasure isn't worth the permanent pain. Think on it, next time you're reaching for the choccies.

- *There are no fat 80-year-olds.* There really is no way around it, mate. There are no doubt a few exceptions here and there. But, look around you. How many

214

80-year-olds do you see carrying the same amount of pud as you have now? Draw the Darwinian deduction. What happened to all the older fat people? Were they hit by a comet? No, they hit the dirt because the Big Macs kept hitting their gut. Lose weight and stay alive. This *has* to be a pretty good argument, no?

- *Only eat when you're hungry. Stop when full. (Or almost full.)* And yes, I know it sounds simple. But for many blokes, like me, when I first came across this mantra, from my niece – who had unaccountably lost a whole heap of weight from one Chrissie to the next – it was like this whole new, *revolutionary* idea to me.

- *When you want to know when you've had enough,* **listen to your stomach, not your eyes**. *You don't have to finish everything on your plate.* I know, this is similar to the one above. But it's a different way of looking at it. Now, like you, I was raised in a house where it was downright rude not to finish everything on your plate. But think on President George Bush Snr. Once he became President in 1988, his first decree was that there would be no more broccoli served on Air Force One, or in the White House, or at any dinner that he was hosting – prompting strong protests from the broccoli farmers of America, who threatened to dump tons of broccoli on the White House lawn. President Bush, the Smarter One, didn't blink. He stared those bastards down! 'I do not like broccoli,' the American President declared. 'And I haven't liked it since I was a little kid and my mother made me eat it. And I'm President of the United

States, and I'm not going to eat any more broccoli!' The point is, even though it is ingrained in you and me to finish what is on our plate, for fear of being rude, and fear of being wasteful, our mothers aren't watching us anymore. We are running this show. And it is actually every bit as wasteful, and more damaging, to eat food we don't actually need.

- *Breakfast like a king, lunch like a prince, dinner like a pauper ...* The oldest one in the book, taught to me by my elder brother Andrew when I was ten years old, and it only took me another 40 years or so to realise its worth. The theme is that if you fill your tank with good healthy food at breakfast – after your ten-hour fast of the night before – then lunch should be no more than a good top-up and dinner a minor top-up.

- *Abs are made in the kitchen, not in the gym.* Yes, you can exercise a lot and feel great, but if you eat a lot of bad food you will still look bad. Bad Food beats Good Gym. Speaking of American presidential politics, I am reminded of the time when the American political savant James Carville appeared on David Letterman's show in the early 1990s. Newly elected President Clinton had made headlines for going jogging three times a week and wearing a tracksuit in the Oval Office. Letterman asked Carville why, if the President kept jogging all the time he, uh, appeared to be, uh, tubby? Carville didn't pause for a beat before he replied: 'Because a Big Mac every day beats jogging three times a week.'

- *It took more than a day to put it on. It will take more than a day to take it off.* Rome wasn't built in a day and neither was your gut. It took time and effort and so will reversing it. It won't happen overnight, but it will happen, if you take action.

- *You'll never regret exercising. But you'll always regret not exercising.* You must know it, yes? When did you ever come back from a run, or the like, feeling anything other than virtuous? And how often have you stayed in, instead, feeling like a slug, and the feeling lasts clear until the next morning?

- *Do not reward yourself with food, you're not a dog . . .* Animals eat when food is presented to them, because they don't know when their next meal is coming. You do. And you know if it's coming from somewhere with Golden Arches in front of it, you are 'rewarding' yourself like a dog and too often eating like a pig. Use your head to make the right decisions, not your gut to make the wrong ones.

- *It's easier to keep up than catch up.* This might seem obvious. But it was a breakthrough for me. Going from obese, to overweight, and then to healthy can be a challenge. The svelte mob of our generation is well up ahead, effortlessly and gracefully – if often ungraciously – loping away into their healthy senior years. And you and I have been stuck with the fatties up the back, with more and more blokes cartwheeling off into the ditch, all around us. We are going to have to *work* to put in extra effort, to catch up. Some parts of changing your

217

diet really can be difficult – otherwise every bastard would do it, no worries, yes? But once you've made the change? It's a piece of piss. When you've caught up with the svelte mob, and loping along at a leisurely pace, it couldn't be easier. You just need to keep on keeping on. And be determined not to fall back.

- *Don't eat sweet.* For what it's worth, this is my encapsulation of Gillespie's general theme, an encapsulation he heartily endorses. If you simply cut sweet things out of your diet, everything else sorts itself out.

- *Real food isn't symmetrical.* Sure, there are exceptions like a perfectly formed banana, I guess. But, generally, if it is square, or rectangular, or perfectly round, it has come to you from a factory, and you shouldn't eat it.

- *The whiter your bread, the quicker you're dead.* White bread has been processed far more than multigrain and brown breads. As a result your body will burn through the energy quicker. Also the process of making white bread reduces its nutritional value, and removes much of the natural fibre.

- *Don't add sugar to anything.* This one should be obvious, but it's worth remembering. If you drink coffee, have it black or white but you don't need a teaspoon of sugar added to it. And don't tell me that you need sugar to make the coffee drinkable. If you don't like coffee until you add sugar, then guess what? *You don't like coffee* – you like sugar. The same is true of tea and anything else with which you might be tempted to put sugar.

• *You blokes, with your bodies, it's like you have inherited a Picasso and yet every day, you throw shit at it!* Good one, isn't it? It was a line used by Sydney medico Dr Adrian Burton, when speaking to corporate audiences. His point was that all of us have inherited this extraordinary *masterpiece* of creation – finely tuned, intricately engineered, and calibrated down to the last degree. It is a blessing beyond measure. And yet we treat it disgracefully, constantly throwing shit at it, in terms of sugar, fat, nicotine, tar, alcohol, total lack of exercise, and all the rest. One reason we do it is that everywhere we look every bastard we can see is doing exactly the same. They're all eating and drinking too much, too, and abusing their bodies in different ways, so we take that as normal, just as we take the bodies that result as normal. But it's not. And we have to stop, clean off our Picassos and let 'em *shine*!

All of the above lines come from here and there, and most of them are well known.

The American health guru Michael Pollan, however, in his 2008 book, *In Defense of Food*, penned a famous credo which, he noted, in just seven words could sum up everything he'd learned about food and health:

'Eat food. Not too much. Mostly plants.'

Wait, wait, wait! There's nothing inherently wrong with meat, Pollan's just saying – and my experience backs it up – that it would likely do you good to eat a little less of it.

And there is no doubt that a unifying feature of just about every healthy long-term eating plan you will come across is that we need to eat heaps more veggies and salad, and less meat – or even no meat at all.

Pollan's fascinating thesis is that we all should refuse to eat anything that comes from the 'food-industrial complex', because it is that very entity which is killing both us and the planet. It means don't eat anything your great-grandmother wouldn't recognise.

That book, and the pithy concept it contained, was so successful that Pollan recently published another book, *Food Rules*, containing 64 equally eloquent lines – or rules, if you will – with the broad theme that by following them, both the reader and the planet could become healthier at once.

Try Rule No. 19: *'If it's a plant, eat it. If it was made in a plant, don't.'*

And look to Rule No. 20: *'It's not food if it arrived through the window of your car.'*

Rule No. 24: *'Eating what stands on one leg [mushrooms and plant foods] is better than eating what stands on two legs [fowl], which is better than eating what stands on four legs [cows, pigs and other mammals].*

On the subject of sugar in food, Rule 35 is very simple: *'Eat sweet foods as you find them in nature.'*

And Rule 36: *'Don't eat breakfast cereals that change the color of the milk.'*

Rule 48. *'Consult your gut.'* Love it! As I write this, the kind flight attendant on QF02 coming back to Sydney from

London has just offered me some no doubt delicious savouries. I consulted my gut. Am I hungry? My gut said no. How could I be, after the omelette I just had in Dubai an hour ago? I declined.

Rule 50. *'The banquet is in the first bite.'* And I love this one, too. Just seven words to contain a whole philosophy. When you and I were young, gormless and gauche, the two key eating pleasures we knew were: eating heaps of sugar and heaps of fat. We didn't savour the flavour, we just whacked it into us. Pollan proposes a new way: savour it, go slow, treasure the pleasure of eating smaller amounts of delicious and healthy food, rather than just piling crap into us.

Anyway, you get the drift. Some of these lines will stick, some won't. The idea is to harness the ones that do, to make positive change.

FOURTEEN

What I know now

'*Any fool can know. The point is to understand . . .*'
Albert Einstein

'*The doctor of the future will give no medicine, but
instead will interest his patients in the care of the
human frame, in diet, and in the cause and prevention
of disease.*'
Thomas Edison

I met this Australian biker once, who, dinkum, could have
stabbed Adolf Hitler, and didn't.

For you see, the great cyclist Edgar 'Dunc' Gray was an
Olympic Gold Medallist at the Los Angeles Olympics in
1932 in the 1000 metre time trial, and so highly regarded by
his fellow athletes and officials of the Australian Olympic

team that in 1936 he was accorded the supreme honour of carrying Australia's flag at the Berlin Olympics.

Which is why, at Berlin's Olympiastadion, on 1 August 1936, for one frozen moment in time, he looked at the pointy end of the spear-like staff that the Australian flag was attached to, looked at Adolf Hitler swanning past just 15 yards away, and in a moment of madness thought that he would probably be doing a very good thing if he just bloody well drove the spear into Hitler's heart and be done with it.

The Australian Olympic team had had jack of Germany by this time, and were beginning to realise what a Fascist state close up really looked like. From the moment they'd arrived for the Games, there seemed to be just a bad feeling in the air, with more Nazi flags displayed everywhere than there were Olympic flags, armed soldiers omnipresent, and the knowledge that the newly constructed Olympic Village they were staying in was going to be – what else but? – an officers' barracks after they left.

What's more, the Australian team couldn't help but notice that the German people generally gave the serious impression of being right into this cove Hitler, that all of Europe and the world was talking about. You'd never believe it if you hadn't seen it with your own eyes, but when the Germans met each other in the street, instead of shaking hands or giving a Teutonic version of 'How ya going?' they would throw their arm out and yell '*Heil Hitler!*' and all that sort of malarkey.

Sure, the Australian Olympic team got into it, too, after a while, and started shouting out at each other 'Hail Mary!'

as they passed each other in the corridor . . . or even 'Haile Selassie!' in reference to the Emperor of Ethiopia then in the news for leading the resistance to an invasion of his country by the absurd little Italian dictator, Benito Mussolini, but the whole thing was a worry all right.

And of course, Gray didn't jab Hitler, something he was still regretting in his Kiama home a good 60 years later when I interviewed him, just before he died. But something else he said to me that day has always stayed with me.

Back in the early 1930s, he had a seminal conversation.

'I particularly remember,' he reminisced, 'a journalist by the name of Harry Gordon told me something very important. He asked me once if I ever weighed myself when I was in good form, and I said "No". He said, "Well, you might find that it will be useful to find out what weight you are, and then try to keep to it, to stop yourself going fat." And you know he was right? The weight and everything go together, see, and if you weigh right, you'll go right. It made a big difference to me, knowing that.'

Do you get it?

This was a bloke who had already won Olympic bronze, had countless Australian titles and was deeply experienced in all matters to do with preparation to ride fast. And yet, even at the age of 25, as one of the fastest cyclists in the world, he hadn't yet grasped a fact that you and I take for granted, as bleeding bloody obvious. Not because he was obtuse, but because the bleeding bloody obvious to us in the 21st century hadn't yet been worked out in the early 1930s, or at least not widely understood at that time.

And I reckon there are many parallels in getting your weight under control. Because I have got interested in the whole thing and have read up on it, and talked to experts, there are things I now get that I had absolutely no clue of before. As a small example, before Test matches with the Wallabies, I drank as little water as possible for three days in the *ludicrous* belief that being a kilo or two lighter because of it would be more beneficial than the damage done by having no water in what was effectively my body's radiator. Before the last Test I played in Australia, I stayed in a super-hot bath that morning, on the reckoning it would soothe my muscles and have me fresh for the match. (It didn't.)

Now, in this field of basic health, with so many claims and counter-claims, surely it is useful to have things we can hang on to? For just as 'fashion changes, but style is eternal', these are facts that are just that – *facts* – which don't change as health fads come and go.

Here is my list of things in the realm of health that should be more widely grasped by you and me and our tubby brethren, but aren't . . .

• **It really is about the sugar.** And, yes, I know I am repeating myself, repeating myself, repeating myself. Twenty-five years ago before a Test against the All Blacks, Bob Dwyer talked to us for 45 minutes about how he wanted us to play, most particularly the back-line. I really concentrated, but could only get five per cent, at best, of what he was on about. Afterwards, I asked the captain Nick Farr-Jones, if *he* understood. 'Ninety-eight per cent of it,' Nick said, 'was run straight, draw your man, and set up the bloke outside you.' BINGO! The essence of it was simple and the rest was just needless complications – the bells and whistles that students of the game get off on, but the rest of us are either bored rigid by or simply don't understand in the first place. In this case, I got it. In the case of our diet, I frankly think, so shoot me, much the same can be said about sugar. If you cut the sugar out of what you put in your mouth, then just about everything else will sort itself out.

- **In terms of losing weight, 80 per cent of it is to do with what you eat, and just 20 per cent the exercise you do.** Yes, I've already detailed that above, but it is a beauty, isn't it? After all is said and done, that gets to the very heart of it. You have got to burn up more pies than you eat. And while you can knock off a pie in seconds – watch me – it can take an *hour* of exercise to burn it off. Yes, you must exercise, on principle, and for the many gains I've discussed in the *Get Moving!* chapter above. But, first up, you need to get on top of what you put in your mouth. This is why they say the best exercise you will ever do is to slowly . . . with your forearms flexed, and your shoulders straight . . . *lower your fork* . . . and now, with both hands on the table . . . *push your chair back.* You've had enough.

- **Your claims that the reason you are overweight is because you have a slow metabolism are nonsense.** Oh come on, you know you have either used that excuse, or heard it, dozens of times! It don't wash, mate. Yes, people have a differing speed of metabolism, but here is the truth: The difference between quick and slow metabolisms is roughly equivalent to the calories in a glass of milk, so don't act like you've been hard done by. (Did you ever see the reality TV show *Survivor*? They would take two dozen people onto an island and they would have to live off very simple food, whatever they could catch, and water, while they competed not to be voted off the island. And you know what? At the end of a month out there the most amazing thing happened! They all lost a hell of a lot of weight. Not a slow metabolism in the bunch once you took away their food and added exercise!) So listen to Mr Tyson. The one thing that legitimate nutritional scientists do not debate is this truth. If you burn more energy than you consume, your body has no other option than to cannibalise itself for energy – and you lose weight. And so to exercise, let's get to it . . .

- **All notions that you can remove flab on a particular part of the body by working on the muscles near and around that part are complete nonsense.** And yes, I know that goes completely counter to all those ads you see on late-night television. As discussed, a lot of those advertorials might not be entirely true . . .

- **We all underestimate what we eat.** Now you may think you are tough on yourself, your own worst critic etc, but there is one area where you and I are both very forgiving: how much we eat. Yes, I know in everyday life we usually have the keen observational powers of Sherlock

Holmes, but when it comes to remembering what we eat, we turn into a very hazy Alan Bond on a particularly forgetful day in the dock. And it's not just us, it's everyone. Study after study shows that if you keep a food diary for a few weeks, you will be reasonably good at estimating what you actually shovelled down your throat during the day. Otherwise, you are as accurate as Blind Freddie, or Fat Freddie. For instance, a 2010 British study of 10,000 dieters by their GPs found that 87 per cent underestimated how much they ate! And these are the figures for dieters! As Richard Gordon, the GP who wrote the *Doctor in the House* books, once observed, everyone who is 'slimming' remembers with 100 per cent clarity each lettuce leaf they bravely ate, but they instantly forget that they transformed into Billy Bunter when they got near a tin of biscuits. It's not a character flaw and it's not just you, it's everyone. When it comes to monitoring how much you eat, you are about as reliable as an Italian train schedule. As Dr Rosemary Stanton says, if everyone in Australia ate only what they claim in surveys, we'd have no fat people. That's one of the reasons your new diet is failing. Here's the next reason . . .

- **Diets don't work.** Or at least they just about never work! Reports really do vary, but it is somewhere between one per cent and five per cent of those who go on a diet actually manage to keep off weight lost in a 12 month period. So stop the nonsense. I repeat one more time: don't go on a diet, *change* your diet.

FIFTEEN

Oh, and by the way

'I think the reward for conformity is that everyone likes you
except yourself.'
Rita Mae Brown, humorist

'The individual has always had to struggle to keep from
being overwhelmed by the tribe. If you try it, you will be
lonely often, and sometimes frightened. But no price is too
high to pay for the privilege of owning yourself . . .'
Friedrich Nietzsche, German philosopher

'Today you are You,
That is truer than true.
There is no one alive
who is Youer than You.'
Dr Seuss, author

Listen, I forgot to mention.

You may have noticed I wear a stupid red rag on my melon? You may have wondered why?

Sometimes, I do too. And there is no doubt that heaps of people think middle-aged men wearing bandanas is just PATHETIC. But I pass this on, on the reckoning that it may be of interest to you, and it might fit into this book under the general title of having a renewed *healthy* outlook.

But seeing as so many people ask for an explanation, here it is.

Let me go back to nigh on three decades ago, when, as mentioned, I was living and playing rugby right in the dead centre of France. (Seriously, if you put the compass point in a map of *L'Hexagone* so it balances, it would go right down the chimney of my farmhouse, just on the fringes of the glorious village of Donzenac.)

And there was this guy, see, not my coach, but the coach of our great rivals, Toulon, a bloke by the name of Daniel Herrero. And he wasn't like the other French coaches with their regulation clothes and their neat haircuts that their mothers could be proud of. He didn't have a neatly trimmed moustache. In fact, he had a big bushy beard, long flowing hair, and a red hairband around the lot to keep it roughly neat – an older extra from *Jesus Christ Superstar*, maybe. He didn't wear suits and ties, or even tracksuits – he wore jeans, held up by flaming red braces.

For he obviously just didn't give a rat's arse what other people thought, because he wasn't trying to fit in with *them*.

It was about what *he* wanted to do, and he was old enough not to care.

And I didn't even know him that well, apart from regularly getting into brawls with his players. One of them jabbed his thumb so deeply into my eye I could see my own brain. It was big.

But I digress, again . . .

Looking back, I guess Daniel Herrero planted a seed in my melon that was a long time in blooming. For the years passed in a flash, the way they do when you pursue your passions, and the next thing I know, I'm rising 50, in Havana, on a family holiday.

At a bazaar by Havana harbour, my eldest son sees a red bandana for sale.

'Dad,' he says, 'you'd look great in that.'

I try it on – he teaches me how to tie it – and I look at myself in the mirror.

'You know, Jake,' I say, 'I reckon I do!'

My second son, Louis, looks, and agrees.

And so does my daughter: 'Daddy, I like it.'

And then the hardest marker of all, my wife – the German judge who doesn't mind holding up the odd 2/10 on the scorecard when it comes to what I am pleased to refer to as my 'fashion choices' – gives her verdict, as the crowd holds its breath.

She slowly nods her head!

'Darling,' says she, warmly, 'that's just *you*.'

A 9.5! In the pike position, with a triple-somersault, she's given it a 9.5! The crowd goes wild.

Sadly, of course – and I really do get this – we are the only five ones that think so. But, so what? I'm over 50, and I'm just past caring.

In the spirit of Daniel Herrero, I don't particularly *like* wearing suits and ties, with short back and sides, so why should I?

And I know, too, many think it's a mid-life crisis, that I should grow out of it. And maybe getting fit and strong and healthy for the first time in yonks is part of the same crisis.

But gee, I enjoy them both!

Don't panic, I'm not suggesting you wear a bandana. But surely there's *something* you've always wanted to do, or wear, but didn't, because of what people might say? As long as it doesn't involve Cheryl from Accounts, and won't hurt you or your family, give it a go!

I thought I'd just leave you with that, as a penultimate thought, mate.

Good luck!

SIXTEEN

In summation

'Gluttony is an emotional escape, a sign something is eating us.'
Peter De Vries, American author

'This is the ultimate aim of quitting sugar: to return to our natural appetite, like when we were young kids. And when you achieve it, Golly, it's food freedom!'
Sarah Wilson, I Quit Sugar For Life

In summary, Just Stop Being a Fat Fuck, OK? (This was the original book title, but my publisher ran screaming from the room.)

Mate, now that we have passed a certain age, the game has changed. Do you remember that fabulous and famous interaction between Prime Minister Paul Keating and Opposition Leader John Hewson back in 1993, when they were jostling for position over the GST? Hewson was for it, and had released his 'Fightback!' package, while Keating was deadset against it.

At the climax of the debate, Hewson roared across the ballot box at Keating: 'If you are so confident about your view of Fightback, why will you not call an early election?'

Keating paused. Licked his lips. *Got him.*

'The answer is, mate,' he smiled, 'because I *want to do you slowly.* There has to be a bit of sport in this for all of us. In the psychological battle stakes, we are stripped down and ready to go. I want to see those ashen-faced performances; I want more of them . . .'

And I, no kidding, feel the same way about life.

I've loved my life for the first half-century on this planet, but I want *more* of it! As I get older, I don't really want to slow down, be on first-name terms with the doctor's receptionist, see my weight get to dangerous levels, watch my blood pressure soar, get gout, suffer the gradual loss of movement of my limbs or the atrophying of my brain as I head off on seeing a bewildering round of specialists. I want to live in my 50s and 60s and into my 70s, 80s and beyond, as a healthy man! More than just growing old disgracefully – if you think the bandana is bad, you ain't seen nothing yet – I want to have the *energy* to do so!

And I have realised that to maximise my chances of staving off the aforementioned, and having the chance to live the way I want, I have to make the changes to the way I live . . . *now.*

I imagine you are in the same position, yes?

But here's the thing.

You and me, mate, we need to *commit* to it, not just engage in a half-arsed, half-involved, I-might-give-this-a-try-to-get-the-missus-off-my-back sort of way. Hopefully, some of the things in this book will have made an impact on you to the point that you really are determined to make that change. But, I repeat, you need to COMMIT.

There's a sign up on the blackboard of the gym I go to which says:

> *Commitment is keeping to something, even though the mood you were in when you made that commitment has passed.*

I like that. If you really are going to do this, you need to set yourself to do it beyond the usual piss-weak day or two – you heard me – that you and I always got to after New Year's.

And, as it happens, I can cite an even better definition of what commitment is.

Way back when, Alan Jones was addressing the Wallabies at a breakfast meeting at the Manly Pacific Hotel, on the need for *commitment* to the game plan in the Test against the All Blacks that afternoon, not mere *engagement*.

In full Churchillian cry, Jones seized on the nearest metaphor to hand to illustrate his point.

'Look at that,' he cried, 'bacon and eggs for breakfast. The chicken was involved, but the pig . . . the pig was *committed*!'

Boom-boom!

(Some Wallabies got it immediately, some didn't twig till about midway through the second half.)

So, too, with this. If you are dinkum about losing weight, sobering up and all the rest, what you have to do is this: face the truth – the elephant in the room is YOU.

Oi! You. Fatty Boomka.

Yes, you, I *am* talking to you . . .

Start . . . now.

Stop eating processed foods. Completely. Wrap your head around this central notion: stop the sugar = stop the hunger.

Get off the piss. Not a little bit, not a lot. *Totally.*

Get your arse moving. Every day, as part of your routine.

Weigh yourself every morning and record it.

After a month, you will be jumping with joy at the results, but still incapable of jumping over the Brownie points you've accumulated from your missus. Spend them wisely.

And *keep going*. Don't be a weak prick and drift back into the old ways, for that is a miserable cliché, just like you and I *used* to be.

We don't do that shit anymore, remember?

We've changed. Our diets. Our lives.

Personally, I have rediscovered what it feels like to be young again. I had dinkum forgotten that feeling – but now I feel so strong, I am dangerous! No kidding, when I did the biography of war heroine Nancy Wake – *aka* the 'White Mouse' – I learned a lesson that has stayed with me since. Although she was a very old woman when I started, all of 90 years old, the same fearless and youthful spirit that was the terror of the Nazis – able to launch ambushes, blow up bridges and all the rest – was *100 per cent intact* inside her frail body. (She and I had quite a few blues early on, until we both came to the conclusion she was ten times the man I would ever be.) The lesson I have learned from this exercise is that not only is the youthful spirit in me, still alive, but I can also reawaken it in my still youthful body! I repeat: I was not, as I thought, old, fat and slow. I was just fat and slow. Now that I have lost the fat, everything else has come good!

And I reckon it will for you, too.

Good luck with it, mate. Let me know how you go.

Acknowledgements

Many people had input into this, none more so than David Gillespie, who was generous from first to last in sharing his knowledge with me, as well as his contacts. I record my deepest gratitude to him. Rory Robertson was equally generous. The journey I was on was precisely the one Rory had headed down a few years ago, and he had much the same attitude as me: how, when this is so easy once you get the hang of it – lose the sugar! – can it be that everyone doesn't know it? He, like Gillespie, proved to be a great intellectual guide, constantly pointing to sources, as to how it all fits together.

Meantime, I regard Dr Robert Lustig as, if not the fount of knowledge on the subject of sugar – as that title perhaps more properly belongs to the late John Yudkin – then at least the largest reservoir, and whenever I was lost I would make my way back to his teachings. I consulted with Dr Lustig on a couple of key points where he put me right, and, at his suggestion, leant heavily on his associate, Professor Alejandro Gugliucci, to make sure my science was correct. Professor Gugliucci could not have been more helpful, and I warmly thank him. Dr John Cummins vetted the manuscript from a purely medical perspective, and has my gratitude.

I also thank the eldest of John Yudkin's sons, Professor Michael Yudkin, himself a biochemist at Oxford University, for vetting my material and ensuring I did the pioneering work of his late, great, father justice.

Ditto Professor Stephen Simpson of Sydney University, who was very helpful. I should note, at this point, it proved impossible to get one expert to agree with all the points raised by all the others, or at least what emphasis should be placed on what aspects of a diet to become healthy as quickly as possible, but that – I have discovered – remains the very nature of nutritional science. The best way, it seemed, was, when differences arose, to defer to those in whose special field it lay. I was careful, too, to get the most highly regarded dietitian in the country, Dr Rosemary Stanton, to look at the manuscript, to ensure that – though she disagrees on a few matters of emphasis and interpretation – my advice remained within the parameters of good nutrition.

In terms of actually putting the book together, it was more of a family affair than any other book I've ever done. As my son Jake had just graduated from Sydney Uni with his Arts degree, and was both interested in the subject and knowledgeable, it was a joy to work together with him doing much of the research, while hauling my kite back to earth when it was flying too wildly, and constantly providing his own insights.

My cousin Angus FitzSimons was also extremely helpful, as he knew from the first exactly what I was trying to achieve with the book, and his oft-humorous input and in-depth research was extremely valuable – most particularly when two, and even three professors gave differing views, and I was trying to see the way forward.

On a lot of the physical movement stuff, I am indebted to brother and sister Shane and Jess Cross, who preside at the gym where I work out and had vast experience and knowledge to call on that they were happy to share. My own brother, David FitzSimons, was wonderful, as always, reading the manuscript from the point of view of 'everyman', and giving cogent feedback.

In terms of living with a man given to excess, few are more experienced than my wife, Lisa, and she was great in helping to frame the book so that what I have learned could – *tap-tap-tap tappity-tap* – be put in terms that others could tap into, too. She edited it from first to last – using skills she'd first honed editing the likes of *Dolly*, *Cleo* and *The Australian Women's Weekly* – made many suggestions and came up with the title, which I love.

My publisher, Alison Urquhart, loved the concept from the first moment I mentioned it to her, and has been wonderfully supportive throughout.

Endnotes

Chapter 1

1 www.abc.net.au/news/2014-02-23/heart-foundation-data-shows-average-weight-increasing/5277850.
2 www.aihw.gov.au/australias-health/2014/ill-health/.

Chapter 3

1 http://www.goodfood.com.au/good-health/the-best-and-worst-diets-2016-three-experts-share-their-verdicts-20160129-gmgwqz.

Chapter 4

1 www.statnews.com/2016/09/12/sugar-industry-harvard-research/.

Chapter 5

1 https://static.diabetesaustralia.com.au/s/fileassets/diabetes-australia/e7282521-472b-4313-b18e-be84c3d5d907.pdf.

Chapter 6

1   A short excerpt on the line in question: https://www.youtube.com/watch?v=HWh1PSQfdK0.

2   www.uncletobys.com.au/products/oats/gourmet-temptations/berrynut.

3   www.opc.org.au/latestnews/mediareleases/pages/breakfast-cereals-up-to-one-third-sugar.aspx#.V6qyiRLU7fY.

4   www.kelloggs.com.au/en_AU/nutri-grain-product.html.

5   www.theage.com.au/lifestyle/diet-and-fitness/popular-kids-cereals-nutrigrain-coco-pops-frosties-and-fruit-loops-more-than-30-per-cent-sugar-20150316-1m0hay.html.

6   https://en.wikipedia.org/wiki/Muesli.

7   www.howmuchsugar.com/resources/Documents/atp.pdf.

8   www.sti.health.gov.au/internet/publications/publishing.nsf/Content/sugar-drinks-toc~sugar-drinks-3-fact-sheets~sugar-drinks-factsheet-3-3-sugar-what-drink.

9   http://shop.coles.com.au/online/national/golden-circle-apple-mango-juice.

10 www.smh.com.au/business/retail/healthy-smoothies-hiding-more-kilojoules-than-a-big-mac-experts-warn-20160112-gm48a0.html.

11 www.news.com.au/lifestyle/food/eat/this-is-what-an-untouched-mcdonalds-happy-meal-looks-like-after-six-years/news-story/08d435d9cbe841c768c03f13c4a7b671.

12 www.fatsecret.com/calories-nutrition/generic/apple-dried-uncooked?portionid=54007&portionamount=100.000.

13 www.sugarscience.org/the-sweet-science-behind-honey.html.

Chapter 7

1   DAA Media Program Quarter Two Report 2010, http://daa.asn.au/wp-content/uploads/2011/05/Quarter_Two_2010_Media_Report.pdf?52640.

2   www.mdpi.com/journal/nutrients/special_issues/carbohydrates.

3   2010 Aged Care Guide Report, https://news.agedcareguide.com.au/2010/06/03/its-not-about-the-sugar/.

4   Abstract of the 'Australian Paradox', www.ncbi.nlm.nih.gov/pubmed/
    22254107.

5   Brand-Miller in a 9 July 2011 interview with *The Australian*. www.
    theaustralian.com.au/news/health-science/a-spoonful-of-sugar-is-
    not-so-bad/story-e6frg8y6-1226090126776.

6   Abstract of the 'Australian Paradox', www.ncbi.nlm.nih.gov/pubmed/
    22254107.

7   http://daa.asn.au/advertising-corporate-partners/program-
    partners/.

8   DAA media release 2009, http://dmsweb.daa.asn.au/files/media%20
    releases/August_09/MR_Breakfast_Week_August09.pdf.

9   http://arinex.com.au/dietitians2014/sponsored-breakfast-seminars.

10 www.eatdrinkpolitics.com/wp-content/uploads/DAAReportEat
    DrinkPolitics.pdf.

11 www.eatdrinkpolitics.com/wp-content/uploads/DAAReport
    EatDrinkPolitics.pdf. See also, http://daa.asn.au/for-the-public/
    diverse-world-of-dietitians-meet-one-here-today/food-industry/
    in-the-spotlight-anne-marie-mackintosh-apd-an/.

12 Leigh Reeve, https://au.linkedin.com/in/leighreeve.

13 ABS interview with *Lateline*, 2016, www.abc.net.au/lateline/content/
    2015/s4442720.htm.

14 www.abc.net.au/news/2016-04-13/the-australian-paradox:-
    experts-hit-out-at-sydney-uni-study/7319518.

15 Background Briefing, ABC Radio National, 2014, excerpt on
    Lateline as above.

16 www.abc.net.au/lateline/content/2015/s4442720.htm.

17 www.australianparadox.com/pdf/nutrients-03-00491-s003.pdf.

18 www.abc.net.au/news/2016-04-13/the-australian-paradox:-experts-
    hit-out-at-sydney-uni-study/7319518.

19 www.abc.net.au/lateline/content/2015/s4442720.htm.

20 www.sbs.com.au/topics/life/health/article/2016/07/06/4-diabetes-
    myths-busted.

21 http://diabetesnsw.com.au/what-is-diabetes/faqs/.

22 Ibid.

23 http://allprices.com.au/fruisana-sweetener-fructose/.

24 *Low GI Diet Diabetes Handbook*, by Professor Jennie Brand-Miller, Kaye Foster-Powell, Professor Stephen Colagiuri, Dr Alan Barclay. https://goo.gl/cBk3MV.

25 www.abc.net.au/lateline/content/2015/s4442720.htm.

26 www.nhs.uk/news/2015/07July/Pages/Sugary-drinks-linked-to-8000-new-diabetes-cases-a-year.aspx.

27 www.mayoclinicproceedings.org/article/S0025-6196(15)00040-3/fulltext.

28 https://web.archive.org/web/20160227102508/http://food healthdialogue.gov.au/interet/foodandhealth/publishing.nsf/Content/D59B2C8391006638CA2578E600834BBD/$File/Resources%20and%20support%20for%20reformulation%20activities.pdf.

29 http://ausfoodnews.com.au/2015/07/22/hitting-the-sweet-spot-australias-sugar-consumption-decline-2.html.

30 www.srasanz.org/sras/news-media-faq/current-news/austra-lian-sugar-consumption-decline.

31 www.abc.net.au/radionational/programs/backgroundbriefing/2014-02-09/5239418#transcript.

32 https://web.archive.org/web/20150717122652/http://sydney.edu.au/research/documents/australian-paradox-report-redacted.pdf.

33 www.sugaraustralia.com.au/Shared/Green%20Pool%20Report%20Media%20Release.pdf

34 http://heartfoundation.org.au/healthy-eating/heart-foundation-tick

35 www.mayoclinicproceedings.org/article/S0025-6196(15)00040-3/fulltext.

36 www.ucsf.edu/news/2015/10/136676/obese-childrens-health-rapidly-improves-sugar-reduction-unrelated-calories.

37 www.news.com.au/finance/sugar-trap-heart-foundation-critics-say-tick-deals-with-nestle-uncle-tobys-mcdonalds-aldi-too-sweet-to-ignore/story-e6frfm1i-1226265842672.

38 http://well.blogs.nytimes.com/2015/09/28/coke-spends-lavishly-on-pediatricians-and-dietitians/?_r=0.

39 www.abc.net.au/news/health/heart-tick-retires-what-worked-what-didn't/7020732.

40 www.heartfoundation.org.au/news/thank-you-tickf.

41 www.smh.com.au/business/consumer-affairs/heinz-in-hot-water-over-shredz-healthy-toddler-snacks-20160620-gpnvr2.html.

42 http://newsroom.heart.org/news/children-should-eat-less-than-25-grams-of-added-sugars-daily.

43 In the quote, 'Alcohol, cigarettes . . .' the ellipsis replaces the word cocaine. I omit in the text because the whole issue of drug law reform is distracting from the thrust of his point here.

44 www.ibtimes.com/nutrition-industry-sold-out-coca-cola-pepsico-kellogg-hershey-other-junk-food-giants-registered.

45 www.nutrition.org/our-members/our-corporate-members/our-sustaining-members/.

46 www.spinwatch.org/index.php/issues/pr-industry/item/69-independence-of-nutritional-information-the-british-nutrition-foundation.

47 http://nutritionnibbles.blogspot.com.au/2010/05/dietitians-of-canada-its-industry.html.

48 www.nutritionaustralia.org/national/resource/nutritionist-or-dietitian.

49 http://davidgillespie.org/the-canadian-heart-foundation-comes-down-hard-on-sugar/.

50 http://davidgillespie.org/the-canadian-heart-foundation-comes-down-hard-on-sugar/.

51 http://bmcmedicine.biomedcentral.com/articles/10.1186/s12916-015-0281-z.

52 www.singjupost.com/bitter-truth-sugar-robert-lustig-full-transcript/4/.

Chapter 8

1 A Big Mac in Australia has 493 calories according to their website https://mcdonalds.com.au/menu/big-mac. The average calories in a bottle of table wine, according to Aus. Calorie and Fat Counter, is 560. Four beers is 560 calories too.

2 Quote from *Drinking: A Love Story* by Caroline Knapp, Dell Publishing, a division of Bantam Doubleday Dell Publishing Group, Inc., 1996.

CHAPTER 10

1   www.blackdoginstitute.org.au/docs/Factsandfiguresaboutmental
    healthandmooddisorders.pdf.
2   www.abs.gov.au/ausstats/abs@.nsf/lookup/33C64022ABB5ECD5
    CA257B8200179437?opendocument.